COMPREHENSIVE CLINICAL GUIDELINES

Essential Insights for Diagnosis, Treatment, and Prescription in Hospital and Clinical Settings

Roy J. Hansen, MD, Ph.D
Devon A. Magnuson, Pharm.D, BCPS

Copyright © 2024 by Roy J. Hansen, MD, Ph.D, and Devon A. Magnuson, Pharm.D, BCPS All rights reserved. No part of this publication may be reproduced, distributed, or transmitted in any form or by any means, without the prior written permission of the copyright holder, except for the use of brief quotations in a review or scholarly work, as permitted under the fair use doctrine.

Preface

The realm of clinical practice is ever-evolving, and healthcare professionals are tasked with the continuous challenge of delivering the highest standard of care to their patients. A key to navigating the complexities of medical practice lies in an informed, systematic approach to diagnosis, treatment, and prescription. This book, COMPREHENSIVE CLINICAL GUIDELINES: Essential Insights for Diagnosis, Treatment, and Prescription in Hospital and Clinical Settings, aims to bridge the gap between theory and practice by providing actionable, evidence-based guidelines to assist clinicians in decision-making at the point of care.

The authors, Dr. Roy J. Hansen, MD, Ph.D, and Dr. Devon A. Magnuson, Pharm.D, BCPS, bring together their extensive backgrounds in clinical medicine and pharmacy to offer a comprehensive resource that covers the critical aspects of patient management across hospital and clinical settings. Dr. Hansen's expertise as a physician and researcher informs the clinical evaluation and diagnostic protocols, while Dr. Magnuson's specialized knowledge in pharmacy and therapeutics ensures that the treatment strategies and prescription recommendations are grounded in both clinical efficacy and pharmacological safety.

This book is designed to be a practical guide for healthcare professionals at every stage of patient care. Whether you are a medical student, resident, nurse, pharmacist, or attending physician, the detailed insights within these pages will equip you with the necessary tools to address the vast array of clinical challenges faced in hospital and outpatient environments. Each chapter is structured to provide both theoretical underpinnings and clear, actionable guidelines for managing common and complex medical conditions, ranging from acute diseases to chronic conditions.

Throughout the text, we have sought to highlight not only the importance of accurate diagnosis and timely treatment but also the significance of individualized patient care. As we all know, each patient is unique, and their management plan should reflect their specific needs, preferences, and circumstances. Thus, this resource emphasizes personalized treatment regimens, including considerations for specific populations, comorbidities, and patient-specific factors.

In addition, this book includes focused sections on prescription best practices, with detailed drug insights designed to enhance the prescriber's ability to select the right medication for the right patient, all while minimizing the risks of adverse drug reactions and promoting therapeutic adherence. Special attention is paid to drug interactions, contraindications, and emerging therapies that will be of value to both the seasoned clinician and the trainee.

The challenges of modern medicine demand an up-to-date, dynamic resource that is both practical and comprehensive. With this in mind, this book integrates the latest clinical guidelines, evidence-based practices, and cutting-edge research findings. Our hope is that it serves as a constant companion to healthcare providers, helping them make informed decisions, improve patient outcomes, and ultimately contribute to the advancement of clinical care.

We would like to express our gratitude to the many professionals and colleagues who have contributed to the development of this work. Their feedback, expertise, and support have been invaluable in making this book both practical and comprehensive. It is our belief that COMPREHENSIVE CLINICAL GUIDELINES will be an essential tool in the clinical decision-making process, empowering healthcare providers to navigate the intricacies of patient care with confidence and precision.

We invite you, the reader, to engage with this text not just as a reference, but as an essential guide that will support your efforts to provide safe, effective, and compassionate care to your patients.

Roy J. Hansen, MD, Ph.D
Devon A. Magnuson, Pharm.D, BCPS
Preface

Table of contents
List of Abbreviations
Glossary
Table of contents
Chapter 1: Key Symptoms and Syndromes
1. Shock
    - Types and Pathophysiology
    - Diagnosis and Early Management
2. Generalized Tonic-Clonic Seizures and Status Epilepticus
    - Identification and Immediate Management
3. Hypoglycemia
    - Symptoms, Causes, and Corrective Actions
4. Fever
    - Evaluation and Management
5. Pain
    - Assessment and Relief Strategies
6. Anemia
    - Signs, Diagnostics, and Treatment
7. Dehydration
    - Grading and Rehydration Strategies
8. Severe Acute Malnutrition
    - Clinical Features and Interventions

Chapter 2: Respiratory Diseases

1. Acute Upper Airway Obstruction
   - Causes and Clinical Signs
   - Rapid Intervention and Airway Patency
2. Rhinitis and Rhinopharyngitis (Common Cold)
   - Viral Origin, Symptoms, and Symptomatic Treatment
3. Acute Sinusitis
   - Inflammatory Process and Treatment Strategies
4. Acute Pharyngitis
   - Viral and Bacterial Causes, Diagnosis, and Treatment
5. Diphtheria
   - Diagnosis, Antitoxin, and Antibiotic Management
6. Other Upper Respiratory Tract Infections
   - Identification and Supportive Care
7. Croup (Laryngotracheitis and Laryngotracheobronchitis)
   - Viral Etiology and Treatment Options
8. Epiglottitis

- Life-Threatening Infection and Emergent Airway Management
9. Bacterial Tracheitis
    - Bacterial Infection, Antibiotics, and Airway Support
10. Otitis
    - Acute and Chronic Otitis Management
11. Acute Otitis Externa
    - Causes and Topical Treatment
12. Acute Otitis Media (AOM)
    - Diagnosis and Antibiotic Management
13. Chronic Suppurative Otitis Media (CSOM)
    - Long-Term Management and Hearing Preservation
14. Whooping Cough (Pertussis)
    - Symptoms, Treatment, and Vaccination
15. Bronchitis
    - Acute and Chronic Forms, Management, and Prevention
16. Acute Bronchitis
    - Viral Causes and Supportive Care
17. Chronic Bronchitis
    - Long-Term Management and Prevention

18. Bronchiolitis
    - Viral Infection in Infants and Supportive Care
19. Acute Pneumonia
    - Pathophysiology, Causes, and Timely Treatment
20. Pneumonia in Children Under 5 Years
    - Risks and Management
21. Pneumonia in Children Over 5 Years and Adults
    - Diagnosis and Treatment Strategies
22. Persistent Pneumonia
    - Management of Non-Resolving Infections
23. Staphylococcal Pneumonia
    - Aggressive Antibiotic Therapy
24. Asthma
    - Chronic Inflammation, Acute and Long-Term Management
25. Acute Asthma Attack
    - Triggers, Bronchodilators, and Corticosteroids
26. Chronic Asthma
    - Long-Term Medication and Lifestyle Management
27. Pulmonary Tuberculosis
    - Diagnosis, Treatment, and Prevention of Spread

Chapter 3: Gastrointestinal Disorders

1. Acute Diarrhea
   - Causes, Symptoms, and Rehydration Strategies
2. Shigellosis
   - Bacterial Infection, Transmission, and Antibiotic Treatment
3. Amoebiasis
   - Parasitic Infection, Diagnosis, and Anti-Amoebic Treatment
4. Disorders of the Stomach and Duodenum
   - GERD, Gastric and Duodenal Ulcers, and Dyspepsia Management
5. Gastro-oesophageal Reflux Disease (GERD)
   - Causes, Symptoms, and Treatment Approaches
6. Gastric and Duodenal Ulcers in Adults
   - Pathophysiology, Risk Factors, and Treatment Protocols
7. Dyspepsia
   - Causes, Differential Diagnosis, and Symptom Management
8. Stomatitis

- Causes, Diagnosis, and Management of Oral Inflammation

9. Oral and Oropharyngeal Candidiasis
   - Diagnosis and Antifungal Treatment of Oral Thrush

10. Oral Herpes
    - Herpes Simplex Virus, Oral Sores, and Antiviral Management

11. Other Infectious Causes
    - Diagnosis and Treatment of Oral and GI Infections

12. Stomatitis from Scurvy (Vitamin C Deficiency)
    - Clinical Presentation and Role of Vitamin C Supplementation

13. Other Lesions Resulting from Nutritional Deficiency
    - Oral Lesions from Vitamin and Mineral Deficiencies and Nutritional Recovery

Chapter 4: Dermatological Conditions

1. Parasitic Infestations
   - Scabies and Lice: Transmission, Clinical Manifestations, and Management
2. Fungal Infections

- Superficial Fungal Diseases: Diagnosis and Antifungal Therapies
3. Bacterial Infections
   - Impetigo, Furuncles, Carbuncles, Erysipelas, Cellulitis, and Cutaneous Anthrax: Pathogenesis and Treatment
4. Endemic Treponematoses
   - Yaws and Pinta: Epidemiology and Therapeutic Interventions
5. Leprosy
   - Mycobacterium Infection: Skin and Systemic Manifestations, Diagnosis, and Control
6. Viral Dermatology
   - Herpes Simplex and Herpes Zoster: Antiviral Treatments and Symptom Management
7. Other Skin Disorders
   - Eczema, Seborrheic Dermatitis, Urticaria, and Pellagra: Pathophysiology, Diagnosis, and Evidence-Based Treatments

Chapter 5: Eye Diseases
1. Xerophthalmia (Vitamin A Deficiency)

- Role of Vitamin A Deficiency in Eye Damage: Prevention and Dietary Improvements

2. Conjunctivitis
   - Causes and Presentation: Differentiating Bacterial, Viral, and Allergic Forms for Tailored Treatment

3. Neonatal Conjunctivitis
   - Infectious Origins and Prompt Intervention to Prevent Complications

4. Viral Epidemic Keratoconjunctivitis
   - Contagion, Supportive Care, and Infection Control Measures

5. Trachoma
   - Chronic Infectious Disease: Prevention and Treatment to Avert Blindness

6. Periorbital and Orbital Cellulitis
   - Superficial vs. Deep Infections: Early Diagnosis and Antibiotic Therapy

7. Other Pathologies
   - Onchocerciasis (River Blindness): Transmission, Diagnosis, and Treatment

- Loiasis: Clinical Presentation and Antiparasitic Therapy
- Pterygium: Prevention and Surgical Intervention

8. Cataract
- Leading Cause of Reversible Blindness: Surgical Correction and Lens Replacement Advances

Chapter 6: Parasitic Diseases

1. Malaria
- Mosquito-borne Disease: Plasmodium Species and Associated Complications

2. Human African Trypanosomiasis (Sleeping Sickness)
- Caused by Trypanosoma Species: Neurological Symptoms and Sleep Disturbances

3. American Trypanosomiasis (Chagas Disease)
- Caused by Trypanosoma : Impact on Heart and Digestive System

4. Leishmaniasis
- Leishmania Parasites: Cutaneous, Mucocutaneous, and Visceral Forms

5. Intestinal Protozoan Infections (Parasitic Diarrhea)
   - Infections from Protozoa like Entamoeba : Gastrointestinal Symptoms
6. Flukes
   - Liver, Lung, and Blood Flukes: Schistosomiasis and Fascioliasis
7. Schistosomiasis
   - Caused by Schistosoma Species: Damage to Liver, Intestine, and Urinary Tract
8. Cestodes (Tapeworms)
   - Intestinal Infections: Nutritional Deficiencies and Abdominal Discomfort
9. Nematode Infections
   - Roundworms: Ascariasis, Trichuriasis, and Strongyloidiasis
10. Filariasis
    - Parasitic Infection: Lymphatic Damage and Elephantiasis
11. Onchocerciasis (River Blindness)
    - Caused by volvulus: Skin and Eye Lesions, Blindness
12. Loiasis

- Caused by Loa loa: Migrating Adult Worms under Skin and Conjunctiva

13. Lymphatic Filariasis (LF)
    - Filarial Worms: Lymphatic System Damage and Elephantiasis

Chapter 7: Bacterial Diseases

1. Bacterial Meningitis
   - Inflammation of the Brain and Spinal Cord Membranes Due to Bacterial Infection
2. Tetanus
   - Infection by Clostridium tetani Leading to Muscle Stiffness and Spasms
3. Enteric Fevers (Typhoid and Paratyphoid)
   - Systemic Infections Caused by Salmonella Species, Resulting in Fever and Gastrointestinal Symptoms
4. Brucellosis
   - Zoonotic Infection from Brucella Species, Causing Fever, Sweats, and Muscle Pain
5. Plague
   - Fatal Infection Caused by Yersinia pestis, Leading to

Fever, Lymph Node Swelling, and Septicemia
6. Leptospirosis
   - Bacterial Infection Transmitted by Animals, Presenting with Flu-like Symptoms
7. Relapsing Fever (Borreliosis)
   - Recurrent Fever Episodes Caused by Borrelia Species
8. Louse-borne Relapsing Fever (LBRF)
   - Transmitted by Lice, Characterized by Recurring High Fever
9. Tick-borne Relapsing Fever (TBRF)
   - Similar to LBRF, but Transmitted by Ticks
10. Eruptive Rickettsioses
    - Diseases Caused by Rickettsia Species, Typically Presenting with Rashes and Fever

Chapter 8: Viral Diseases
1. Measles
   - Contagious Viral Infection with Fever, Rash, and Respiratory Symptoms
2. Poliomyelitis

- Viral Disease Affecting the Nervous System, Causing Paralysis

3. Rabies
   - Fatal Viral Encephalitis Transmitted by Animal Bites

4. Viral Hepatitis
   - Infections Leading to Liver Inflammation and Complications

5. Dengue
   - Mosquito-borne Viral Illness with Fever, Rash, and Potential Hemorrhagic Manifestations

6. Viral Hemorrhagic Fevers
   - Severe, Often Fatal Illnesses, Including Ebola and Marburg

7. HIV Infection and AIDS
   - Progressive Disease Weakening the Immune System, Increasing Susceptibility to Infections and Cancers

Chapter 9: Genito-Urinary Diseases

1. Nephrotic Syndrome in Children
   - Characterized by Protein Loss, Swelling, and Complications

2. Urolithiasis
   - Formation of Urinary Tract Stones, Causing Pain and Symptoms
3. Acute Cystitis
   - Bladder Infection with Painful Urination and Frequent Urges
4. Acute Pyelonephritis
   - Kidney Infection Presenting with Fever, Flank Pain, and Urinary Symptoms
5. Acute Prostatitis
   - Prostate Gland Infection with Pain, Fever, and Urinary Difficulties
6. Genital Infections
   - Bacterial, Viral, and Fungal Infections Affecting the Genital Region
7. Urethral Discharge
   - Common Symptom of Urethral Infections or Inflammation
8. Abnormal Vaginal Discharge
   - Indicators of Infection or Reproductive Health Issues
9. Genital Ulcers

- Painful Sores Caused by Infections like Herpes or Syphilis
10. Lower Abdominal Pain in Women
    - Pain Related to Reproductive Organs
11. Upper Genital Tract Infections (UGTI)
    - Infections Affecting the Uterus and Fallopian Tubes
12. Venereal Warts
    - Growths Caused by Human Papillomavirus (HPV) on the Genitals
13. Major Genital Infections (Summary)
    - Overview of Significant Genital Infections
14. Abnormal Uterine Bleeding (In the Absence of Pregnancy)
    - Irregular Uterine Bleeding Linked to Hormonal Imbalances or Structural Abnormalities

Chapter 10: Medical and Minor Surgical Procedures
1. Dressings
    - Techniques for Proper Wound Dressing to Promote Healing
2. Treatment of Simple Wounds

- Guidelines for Cleaning and Treating Minor Wounds
3. Burns
    - Management Strategies and Classification of Burns
4. Cutaneous Abscess
    - Approaches for Draining and Managing Skin Abscesses
5. Pyomyositis
    - Treatment of Bacterial Infections in Muscle Tissue
6. Leg Ulcers
    - Care Strategies for Managing Chronic or Acute Leg Ulcers
7. Necrotizing Infections of the Skin and Soft Tissues
    - Urgent Intervention for Severe Infections Requiring Surgical Debridement
8. Venomous Bites and Stings
    - Management of Venomous Animal Bites and Stings, Including Antivenom Use
9. Dental Infections
    - Approaches to Treating Oral Infections, Including

Abscesses and Gum Infections
List of Abbreviations
1. ABG - Arterial Blood Gas
2. ACE - Angiotensin-Converting Enzyme
3. ADA - American Diabetes Association
4. AIDS - Acquired Immunodeficiency Syndrome
5. BUN - Blood Urea Nitrogen
6. BP - Blood Pressure
7. CBC - Complete Blood Count
8. CCU - Coronary Care Unit
9. CT - Computed Tomography
10. DVT - Deep Vein Thrombosis
11. ECG - Electrocardiogram
12. ED - Emergency Department
13. GFR - Glomerular Filtration Rate
14. HIV - Human Immunodeficiency Virus
15. ICU - Intensive Care Unit
16. IV - Intravenous
17. LFT - Liver Function Test
18. MRI - Magnetic Resonance Imaging
19. NSAID - Non-Steroidal Anti-Inflammatory Drug
20. OPD - Outpatient Department
21. OT - Occupational Therapy

22. PCO2 - Partial Pressure of Carbon Dioxide
23. PE - Pulmonary Embolism
24. PID - Pelvic Inflammatory Disease
25. RBC - Red Blood Cell
26. SOB - Shortness of Breath
27. TIBC - Total Iron-Binding Capacity
28. UA - Urinalysis
29. URI - Upper Respiratory Infection
30. WBC - White Blood Cell

Chapter 1
Key Symptoms and Syndromes
This chapter examines a range of critical symptoms and syndromes that frequently arise in clinical practice, emphasizing their recognition and early management:
Shock: Reviews its types, pathophysiology, and the urgency of prompt diagnosis and treatment to mitigate organ damage and improve survival.
Generalized Tonic-Clonic Seizures and Status Epilepticus: Focuses on identifying and managing prolonged or recurrent seizures to prevent neurological complications.

Hypoglycemia: Highlights the symptoms, causes, and immediate corrective actions to avoid severe outcomes.
Fever: Discusses its role as a common indicator of infection or inflammation and approaches for evaluation and management.
Pain: Covers its assessment, types, and strategies for effective relief tailored to the underlying cause.
Anemia: Details the signs, diagnostic considerations, and treatment options for this widespread condition.
Dehydration: Outlines the signs, severity grading, and rehydration strategies to restore fluid balance.
Severe Acute Malnutrition: Examines its clinical features, associated risks, and critical nutritional and medical interventions.
Shock: Comprehensive Overview and Evidence-Based Management
Definition and Impact
Shock is a critical condition characterized by inadequate tissue perfusion and insufficient oxygen delivery to meet cellular demands. If not promptly

diagnosed and treated, it can result in cellular damage, organ failure, and high mortality rates.

Clinical Features of Shock

General Signs:

Suspect shock in patients with clinical signs of tissue hypoperfusion, including:

Skin: Pallor, mottling, sweating, cold extremities, or capillary refill time (CRT) ≥ 3 seconds.

Cardiovascular: Weak radial pulse, low or narrowing pulse pressure, and hypotension (often a late sign, especially in children).

Pulmonary: Tachypnea, dyspnea.

Renal: Oliguria (<0.5–1 mL/kg/hour) or anuria.

Neurological: Anxiety, agitation, confusion, altered mental status.

Signs in Children:

Hypotension is a late and unreliable sign in children. Early indicators include:

Marked lower limb temperature gradient.

Weak radial pulses.

Severe tachycardia.

Types of Shock and Specific Clinical Features

1. Distributive Shock

Pathophysiology: Severe vasodilation and increased capillary permeability leading to abnormal blood distribution.
Subtypes and Features:
Anaphylactic Shock:
Symptoms: Skin or mucosal involvement (urticaria, swelling), respiratory distress, and hypotension.
Risk Factors: Recent allergen exposure (e.g., food, stings, medications).
Septic Shock:
Signs: Fever or hypothermia, altered mental status, persistent hypotension despite fluid resuscitation.
Risk Factors: Infection, recent surgery, immunodeficiency.
2. Cardiogenic Shock
Pathophysiology: Pump failure of the heart leading to inadequate cardiac output.
Features:
Symptoms: Chest pain, dyspnea, arrhythmias, valvular murmurs.
Risk Factors: History of cardiac disease or acute cardiac events.
3. Hypovolemic Shock
Pathophysiology: Loss of intravascular fluid, either through direct fluid loss or sequestration.

Features:
Hemorrhagic: External or internal bleeding with signs of hypotension.
Non-Hemorrhagic: Dry mucosa, sunken eyes, decreased jugular venous pressure, mental status changes.
Risk Factors: Trauma, severe diarrhea, or vomiting.
4. Obstructive Shock
Pathophysiology: Physical obstruction of blood flow to or from the heart.
Features:
Pulmonary Embolism: Chest pain, hypoxia, tachypnea.
Tension Pneumothorax: Tracheal deviation, reduced breath sounds, raised jugular venous pressure (JVP).
Cardiac Tamponade: Pulsus , muffled heart sounds, raised JVP.
Management Strategies
Primary Objectives:
1. Restore tissue perfusion.
2. Normalize vital signs (CRT, SpO_2, BP).
3. Maintain urine output >0.5–1 mL/kg/hour in adults and children.
Initial Steps:

Call for Help: Initiate management promptly, even if the shock type is unclear.

ABC Assessment: Ensure airway, breathing, and circulation stabilization.

Positioning: Lay patient supine unless contraindicated (e.g., spinal trauma or anaphylaxis requiring sitting).

Monitoring:

Regularly measure urine output, BP, CRT, heart rate, respiratory rate, oxygen saturation, and mental status.

Perform targeted diagnostic tests, including blood cultures, glucose, and hematologic parameters.

Type-Specific Management

1. Anaphylactic Shock:

Epinephrine IM: Administer immediately into the mid-anterolateral thigh. Adjust dose according to age.

Airway Support: Oxygen at 10–15 L/min and prepare for intubation if needed.

Adjuncts: Corticosteroids (e.g., prednisolone) for prolonged reactions.

2. Septic Shock:

Fluid Resuscitation:

Adults: 500 mL boluses of Ringer's lactate (RL).
Children: 10 mL/kg rapid infusions.
Antibiotics: Administer broad-spectrum antibiotics within one hour of presentation, tailored based on local resistance patterns.

3. Cardiogenic Shock:
Targeted Interventions: Address underlying arrhythmias, myocardial infarction, or valve dysfunction. Inotropes may be required to enhance cardiac output.

4. Hypovolemic Shock:
Fluids and Blood Products: Administer isotonic crystalloids or blood products based on the type of fluid loss.

5. Obstructive Shock:
Tension Pneumothorax: Immediate needle decompression followed by chest tube insertion.
Cardiac Tamponade: Perform pericardiocentesis.

On-Going Care
Perform regular reassessments (every 10 minutes initially).
Continue nutritional support, emphasizing enteral feeding when possible.

Monitor for fluid overload, especially in vulnerable populations (e.g., elderly, malnourished).

Key Points for Clinical Practice

Early recognition and rapid intervention are essential to prevent irreversible organ damage.

Tailor fluid and pharmacological interventions to the specific type and underlying cause of shock.

Multidisciplinary collaboration is vital for optimal patient outcomes.

Overview of Shock Management and Protocols

Cardiogenic Shock

Cardiogenic shock occurs when the heart fails to pump blood effectively, leading to decreased tissue perfusion. Management includes prompt initiation of vasopressors or inotropes, oxygen therapy, and addressing underlying cardiac issues like acute myocardial infarction or arrhythmias. Advanced life support (ALS) protocols should guide arrhythmia treatment where applicable. Critical care monitoring is essential to ensure hemodynamic stability.

Hypovolemic Shock

1. Non-Hemorrhagic Hypovolemic Shock

Non-hemorrhagic causes, such as severe dehydration or fluid losses due to burns, require cautious fluid replacement.

Adults: Start with 250–500 mL of Ringer's Lactate (RL) solution over 30 minutes.

Adjust subsequent fluids based on patient assessments, such as urine output, mental status, and oxygen saturation.

2. Hemorrhagic Hypovolemic Shock

The primary goal is to prevent the lethal trauma triad: hypothermia, acidosis, and coagulopathy.

Administer blood products as soon as available, halting RL once transfusion starts.

Fluid management protocols:

Children under 20 kg: 20 mL/kg of whole blood.

Adults and children ≥20 kg: Transfuse one adult unit of whole blood.

If blood is delayed, administer RL cautiously:

Children: 20 mL/kg as a rapid bolus.

Adults: 250–500 mL rapidly, repeat as necessary.
Measures like warming blankets and heated IV fluids are crucial.
For trauma within three hours, administer tranexamic acid (TXA):
Children: 15 mg/kg slow IV (max 1 g).
Adults: 1 g slow IV.

Obstructive Shock

Temporary stabilization should include fluid administration under strict monitoring to avoid overload:
Adults: 100–250 mL RL over 30 minutes.
Determine cause and initiate definitive interventions:
Pulmonary embolism: Anticoagulation and/or thrombolysis.
Tension pneumothorax: Immediate needle decompression, followed by chest tube insertion.
Cardiac tamponade: Perform pericardiocentesis.

Airway and Breathing Management

In severe cases, ensure airway patency and oxygenation:

Complete airway obstruction: Endotracheal intubation or cricothyroidotomy.
Respiratory failure: Consider non-invasive or mechanical ventilation.

Circulation Management

Vasopressors are essential if fluid resuscitation fails to achieve adequate blood pressure or tissue perfusion:

1. Norepinephrine (NE) – First-line for adults:

Dilution: Add 2 mL (4 mg) to 38 mL of 0.9% saline for a 0.1 mg/mL solution.

Initiate at 0.1 µg/kg/min, titrating every 10 minutes initially, then hourly, based on clinical objectives.

Maximum rate: 1 µg/kg/min.

2. Epinephrine (EPN) – First-line for children:

Dilution: Add 2 mL (2 mg) to 38 mL of 0.9% saline for a 0.05 mg/mL solution.

Follow a similar titration protocol as norepinephrine.

When stopping vasopressors, reduce dosages gradually to avoid abrupt cardiovascular decompensation.

Fluid Administration Protocols by Age Group
Fluid resuscitation varies depending on age:
Infants (<1 year): 30 mL/kg over 1 hour, then 70 mL/kg over 5 hours.
Children 1–14 years: 30 mL/kg over 30 minutes, then 70 mL/kg over 2.5 hours.
Adolescents ≥15 years and adults: 250–500 mL rapidly, with total fluids adjusted up to 70 mL/kg over 2.5 hours.
Critical Monitoring and Investigations
Continuous monitoring of vitals and laboratory parameters, such as potassium, magnesium, calcium, and phosphate, is essential. Imaging and advanced diagnostic tests, including point-of-care ultrasound (POCUS), should guide further management, provided they are performed by trained professionals.
Special Considerations
1. Postpartum Hemorrhage: Refer to obstetric care guidelines for management.
2. Trauma: Apply tourniquets with care, aiming for surgical

intervention within one hour. Extended tourniquet use (>6 hours) requires specialized surgical management.

3. Anaphylaxis: Use intramuscular epinephrine, titrating vasopressors if shock persists after three doses.

Footnotes for Contextual Understanding

Hypotension: Defined as SBP <90 mmHg or MAP <65 mmHg.

Fluid preferences: Crystalloids are recommended; avoid colloids like albumin.

Calculations for infusion rates must account for weight and drug concentration to prevent overdose or inadequate dosing.

References

1. Houston, K. A., George, E. C., & Maitland, K. (2018). Implications for pediatric shock management in resource-constrained settings: Insights from the FEAST trial. Critical Care, 22(1), 119.

2. Cecconi, M., De Backer, D., Antonelli, M., et al. (2014). Consensus on circulatory shock and hemodynamic monitoring: A Task Force Report from the European Society of Intensive

Care Medicine. Intensive Care Medicine, 40(12), 1795-1815.
3. Cardona, V., Ansotegui, I. J., Ebisawa, M., et al. (2020). World Allergy Organization anaphylaxis guidance 2020. World Allergy Organization Journal, 13(10), 100472.
4. Singer, M., Deutschman, C. S., Seymour, C. W., et al. (2016). The Third International Consensus Definitions for Sepsis and Septic Shock (Sepsis-3). JAMA, 315(8), 801-810.
5. Richey, S. L. (2007). Tourniquets for the control of traumatic hemorrhage: A comprehensive review of the literature. World Journal of Emergency Surgery, 2, 28.
6. Resuscitation Council UK. (2021). Emergency treatment of anaphylaxis: Guidelines for healthcare providers. [Accessed May 31, 2023]. Retrieved from
7. Evans, L., Rhodes, A., Alhazzani, W., et al. (2021). Surviving Sepsis Campaign: International guidelines for the management of sepsis and septic shock (2021). Intensive Care Medicine, 47(11), 1181-1247.

Generalized Tonic-Clonic Seizures and Convulsive Status Epilepticus

Generalized tonic-clonic seizures involve sudden, involuntary movements affecting both sides of the body, accompanied by impaired consciousness or loss of awareness. These episodes arise due to abnormal electrical activity in the brain.

Key Characteristics:

Duration: Most seizures last less than five minutes and resolve spontaneously. They can occur as isolated events or recur.

In children: Seizures often occur during febrile episodes without underlying neurological causes, referred to as febrile seizures.

Status epilepticus (SE): A seizure lasting more than five minutes or multiple seizures within five minutes without regaining baseline consciousness is classified as SE. This is a medical emergency requiring immediate intervention, as prolonged seizures increase the risk of irreversible brain damage and mortality.

Pregnancy/Postpartum Period: Seizures during these phases may indicate eclampsia and require prompt obstetric evaluation.

Clinical Presentation

During a Seizure:

Tonic phase: Prolonged muscle contractions, including respiratory muscles, leading to rigidity.

Clonic phase: Rhythmic jerking of the limbs.

Accompanying symptoms: Cyanosis, difficulty breathing, and involuntary urination.

Postictal Phase (Recovery):

Common symptoms include fatigue, confusion, headache, temporary memory loss, and occasional focal neurological deficits.

Recovery typically occurs within 30–60 minutes but can vary.

First Aid Measures

General Steps:

1. Note the time and seek help immediately.
2. Ensure safety by protecting the individual from falls and loosening restrictive clothing.
3. Positioning: Place the person on their side (recovery position) to prevent aspiration. Avoid inserting objects into their mouth.

4. Manage hypoglycemia: If blood glucose cannot be checked, administer glucose as a precaution.
5. Oxygenation: Administer oxygen if hypoxia is suspected.
6. In cases of suspected febrile seizures, address the fever promptly.

Special Considerations:
In adults with a history of alcohol use, administer thiamine (100 mg IV infusion) concurrently with glucose to address potential vitamin B1 deficiency.
Monitor seizure activity closely to determine the need for further interventions.

Febrile Seizures in Children
Febrile seizures typically occur in children aged 6 months to 5 years during a fever without signs of central nervous system infection or metabolic abnormalities.

Types:
Simple Febrile Seizures: Single generalized episode lasting less than 15 minutes without recurrence within 24 hours.
Low risk of subsequent epilepsy.

Treatment: Observe until full recovery, manage fever, and reassure caregivers.

References

1. Lowenstein DH, Bleck T, Macdonald RL. A call for redefining the criteria of status epilepticus. Epilepsia. 1999;40(1):120-122.
2. Brophy GM, Bell R, Claassen J, et al. Comprehensive guidelines for assessing and managing status epilepticus. Neurocritical Care. 2012;17:3-23.
3. Pottkämper JCM, Hofmeijer J, Van Waarde JA, Van Putten MJAM. Insights into the postictal state: Current knowledge and gaps. Epilepsia. 2020;61(6):1045-1061. https://doi.org/10.1111/epi.16519
4. Steering Committee on Quality Improvement and Management, Subcommittee on Febrile Seizures. Clinical practice guidelines for the prolonged management of children with simple febrile seizures. Pediatrics. 2008;121(6):1281-1286.

Hypoglycemia: Overview, Diagnosis, and Management

Hypoglycemia is characterized by abnormally low blood glucose levels. If left untreated, severe hypoglycemia can result in life-threatening complications or irreversible neurological damage.

Key Points for Clinical Assessment

Blood Glucose Monitoring: Blood glucose levels should be promptly measured in patients exhibiting symptoms of hypoglycemia. When glucose measurement is unavailable, empiric administration of glucose or other accessible sugars is recommended.

Symptoms in Unconscious or Seizing Patients: Hypoglycemia should always be a consideration in individuals presenting with impaired consciousness (lethargy or coma) or seizures.

For neonates, specific diagnostic and treatment protocols are detailed in the Essential Obstetric and Newborn Care guide by MSF.

Clinical Presentation

Hypoglycemia often manifests rapidly with a range of non-specific symptoms, including:

Mild Symptoms: Hunger, fatigue, pallor, anxiety, and sweating.

Severe Symptoms: Tremors, tachycardia, blurred vision, confusion, difficulty speaking, seizures, lethargy, or coma.

Diagnosis

Confirmatory Testing: A capillary blood glucose test (using reagent strips) can confirm hypoglycemia.

Symptom Resolution: In the absence of diagnostic tools, a rapid improvement of symptoms following glucose administration serves as confirmation.

Symptomatic Treatment

Immediate Relief: Oral sugar intake typically alleviates symptoms within 15 minutes. Neurological symptoms generally improve shortly after intravenous (IV) glucose administration.

Follow-Up Testing: Blood glucose levels should be reassessed 15 minutes post-treatment. If levels remain low, repeat glucose administration based on the patient's condition.

If there is no improvement after appropriate glucose

administration, alternative diagnoses should be explored, such as severe infections (e.g., malaria, meningitis), epilepsy, alcohol intoxication, or adrenal insufficiency in pediatric cases.

Post-Stabilization Care

Administer a meal or snack rich in complex carbohydrates.

Monitor the patient for several hours post-recovery to prevent recurrence.

Blood Glucose Thresholds

Non-Diabetic Patients: Hypoglycemia is defined as <3.3 mmol/L (<60 mg/dL); severe hypoglycemia is <2.2 mmol/L (<40 mg/dL).

Diabetic Patients on Treatment: Blood glucose <3.9 mmol/L (<70 mg/dL).

Treatment Guidelines

1. Conscious Patients:

Children: A teaspoon of sugar dissolved in water, 50 mL of fruit juice, maternal or therapeutic milk, or 10 mL/kg of 10% glucose administered orally or via nasogastric tube.

Adults: 15–20 g of sugar (e.g., 3–4 sugar cubes) or a sugary beverage like soda or fruit juice.

2. Patients with Impaired Consciousness or Seizures:
Children: 2 mL/kg of 10% glucose administered slowly over 2–3 minutes via IV.
Adults: 1 mL/kg of 50% glucose administered slowly over 3–5 minutes via IV.
If the patient does not regain full consciousness after severe hypoglycemia, frequent monitoring of blood glucose levels is essential.
Aetiological Treatment
1. Non-Diabetic Causes:
Address underlying conditions, such as severe malnutrition, neonatal sepsis, malaria, or alcohol intoxication.
Modify or discontinue medications known to induce hypoglycemia (e.g., quinine, pentamidine, beta-blockers).
Administer glucose with IV quinine to prevent hypoglycemia when treating malaria.
2. Diabetic Patients:
Ensure regular meal consumption and adjust carbohydrate intake as needed.
Modify insulin doses based on blood glucose monitoring and physical activity.

Reevaluate oral antidiabetic medications to avoid potential drug interactions.

Preparation of Glucose Solutions

For facilities without pre-made 10% glucose solution, prepare the solution by removing 100 mL of 5% glucose from a 500 mL container and replacing it with 50 mL of 50% glucose. This yields 450 mL of 10% glucose solution.

Reference

1. American Diabetes Association. Standards of Care in Diabetes—2023 Abridged for Primary Care Providers. Clinical Diabetes. 2022;41(1):4-31. https://doi.org/10.2337/cd23-as01

Fever Management and Diagnosis

Definition:

Fever is defined as an axillary temperature greater than 37.5°C. It is commonly associated with infections but may also indicate other serious conditions. A thorough clinical evaluation is essential to identify the cause of the fever and determine appropriate treatment.

Clinical Features of Severe Illness

In a febrile patient, first, assess for signs of serious illness. If the patient appears critically ill, or if symptoms suggest a severe infection, immediate medical attention is needed. Common signs of severe illness include:

Petechial or purpuric rashes, meningeal symptoms, heart murmurs, severe abdominal pain, and dehydration.

In cases of severe bacterial infection or sepsis, look for signs such as altered consciousness, rapid heart rate, low blood pressure, rapid breathing, respiratory distress, or seizures. In infants, a bulging fontanel may be observed.

Symptoms of circulatory impairment or shock include weak pulses, low blood pressure, and diminished blood circulation to vital organs.

Possible Causes Based on Symptoms

Fever accompanied by specific symptoms can help identify the underlying cause:

Meningitis or severe malaria may present with meningeal signs or seizures.

Appendicitis, peritonitis, or amoebic liver abscess can cause abdominal pain and signs of peritoneal irritation.
Gastroenteritis or enteric fever may cause diarrhea and vomiting.
Viral hepatitis can present with jaundice and an enlarged liver.
Pneumonia, measles, or tuberculosis may present with a persistent cough.
Orbital cellulitis may cause eyelid erythema, eye pain, and swelling.
Otitis media is suggested by ear pain and a red tympanic membrane.
Mastoiditis may cause swelling behind the ear.
Streptococcal pharyngitis or diphtheria may cause a sore throat with enlarged lymph nodes.
Oral herpes may cause vesicular lesions on the lips and oral mucosa.
Urinary tract infections often cause dysuria, urinary frequency, and back pain.
Cellulitis or necrotizing soft tissue infections present with red, warm, and painful skin.

Osteomyelitis or septic arthritis can cause joint pain and difficulty walking.

Viral hemorrhagic fevers, such as dengue or chikungunya, can cause a rash, bleeding, and joint pain.

In cases of persistent fever, especially when the patient is severely ill, consider the possibility of HIV infection or tuberculosis.

Diagnostic Workup

In evaluating a febrile patient, particularly those with severe symptoms, a thorough diagnostic workup is crucial:

In malaria-endemic regions, a rapid diagnostic test for malaria should be performed.

For children, tests such as urine dipstick, urine culture, blood cultures, and full blood count (FBC) are recommended. A lumbar puncture (LP) should be considered if meningeal signs are present or if there is suspicion of severe bacterial infection or sepsis.

If respiratory distress or signs of severe infection are evident, a chest X-ray may be necessary.

Blood cultures and FBC are advised for persistent fever or when signs of severe infection are present.

Treatment Approach

1. Malaria: If malaria is diagnosed, treatment should begin promptly as outlined in the malaria guidelines.
2. Empiric Antibiotics: For severe infections or suspected sepsis, start empiric antibiotics immediately, adjusting them once the source of infection is confirmed.
3. If no clear source of infection is found, and the patient is stable, hospitalization may be required for further investigation and observation.

Symptomatic Management

Antipyretics can improve comfort but do not prevent complications such as febrile seizures. Paracetamol (acetaminophen) is commonly used for fever control. For children aged 3 months to 12 years, a typical dose is 5–10 mg/kg every 3–4 hours, with a maximum daily dose of 30 mg/kg. For adults and children over 12, doses of 200–400 mg

every 3–4 hours are appropriate, not exceeding 1200 mg daily.
Ibuprofen is also an option for reducing fever, with dosing similar to paracetamol, though it should be used cautiously in certain cases, such as in viral infections where bleeding risks are increased.

Prevention and Management of Complications

Hydration: Ensure the patient remains well-hydrated. For infants, continue breastfeeding. Monitor for signs of dehydration, especially in children.

Avoid Cold Compresses: Do not wrap children in wet towels or cold cloths, as this can increase discomfort and may lead to hypothermia.

Pregnant Women and Breastfeeding Mothers: Only paracetamol should be used in these populations. Avoid other antipyretics like ibuprofen or acetylsalicylic acid (ASA) in cases of viral hemorrhagic fevers, such as dengue, due to the risk of bleeding.

Special Considerations

In malnourished children, further evaluation and specialized care for severe acute malnutrition are critical.

Patients with sickle cell disease require specific management due to their increased vulnerability to infections and related complications.

Conclusion:

Management of fever involves identifying the cause, treating infections promptly, and providing symptomatic relief. Vigilant monitoring and appropriate testing are essential, particularly for young children, the elderly, and those with underlying conditions. Immediate empiric treatment may be necessary for severe cases, while further investigation should guide subsequent management.

Pain Management Overview

Pain arises from various pathological processes and is uniquely expressed by each individual, influenced by factors such as age and cultural background. It remains a subjective experience, meaning that only the patient can accurately assess the level of pain they are experiencing.

Therefore, consistent and systematic pain assessment is essential for effective treatment.

Clinical Features and Pain Assessment

The evaluation of pain involves gathering information through history-taking and clinical examination, which aids in establishing an etiological diagnosis and guiding treatment. Key components in pain assessment include:

Pain Evaluation Scales: Different scales are employed based on patient age and cognitive ability. The Simple Verbal Scale (SVS) is used for children over 5 years and adults to assess pain intensity. For younger children, scales such as the FLACC (Face, Legs, Activity, Cry, Consolability) or NFCS (Neonatal Facial Coding System) are used for observational assessments.

Pain Characteristics: The nature of pain—whether sudden, intermittent, or chronic, as well as its onset during rest, movement, or specific activities—provides important insights into its cause.

Descriptions of pain, such as burning, cramping, or spasmodic pain, can also assist in diagnosis.

Aggravating or Relieving Factors: Understanding what worsens or alleviates the pain is crucial, including any associated systemic signs such as fever, weight loss, or other underlying conditions.

Types of Pain

1. Nociceptive Pain: Often presents as acute pain and is commonly linked to visible causes such as post-surgical pain, burns, or trauma. Neurological examinations typically show no abnormalities, and treatment is often standardized.

2. Neuropathic Pain: Arises from nerve lesions or damage (e.g., following trauma, ischemia, or infections like shingles). This type of pain is usually chronic and may present as persistent discomfort with intermittent sharp, electric shock-like sensations. Neuropathic pain can result from conditions like neural compression, post-amputation pain, or conditions affecting the central nervous system.

3. Mixed Pain: Seen in complex cases, such as cancer or HIV, and requires a more comprehensive management approach.

Pain Intensity and Management
Pain severity is categorized as follows:
No Pain (Score 0)
Mild Pain (Score 1)
Moderate Pain (Score 2)
Severe Pain (Score 3)
For children aged 2 months to 5 years, the FLACC scale evaluates pain based on facial expression, limb activity, and other observable behaviors. For infants younger than 2 months, the NFCS scale is used to gauge pain based on facial expressions, with a score of 2 or more indicating significant pain.

Treatment Approaches
Pain management depends on the type, intensity, and underlying cause of the pain:
1. For Nociceptive Pain: The World Health Organization (WHO) suggests a three-step analgesic ladder for treatment:
Step 1: Non-opioid analgesics like paracetamol or NSAIDs.
Step 2: Mild opioids, such as codeine or tramadol, often

combined with non-opioid analgesics.
Step 3: Strong opioids, primarily morphine, combined with non-opioid medications.
2. Symptomatic Treatment: If no specific cause is found or if the condition is not curable, pain management is symptomatic.
Analgesic Dosing
Mild Pain: Paracetamol and/or NSAIDs may be used.
Moderate Pain: A combination of Paracetamol, NSAIDs, and mild opioids such as tramadol or codeine.
Severe Pain: Strong opioids like morphine combined with paracetamol or NSAIDs.
Analgesics should be prescribed and administered regularly, rather than on demand, for effective pain control. Oral analgesics should be preferred when possible, and treatment should be tailored based on the patient's response to pain management.
Special Considerations for Pediatric Pain Management
Children's pain management requires adjustments in medication dosage based on age

and weight. For example, paracetamol dosage varies for infants and children, with oral doses typically ranging from 10 mg/kg every 6 to 8 hours to 1g every 6 hours for older children and adults.

Morphine Use and Safety

Morphine is highly effective for severe pain but must be used cautiously due to the risk of respiratory depression, which can be fatal in overdose situations. Doses should be gradually increased, with careful monitoring of respiratory rates, particularly in children. If respiratory depression occurs, naloxone may be administered as an antidote.

Furthermore, opioids like morphine and codeine commonly cause constipation, which necessitates the prescription of a laxative for long-term opioid use.

Conclusion

Effective pain management is crucial for patient care, and it hinges on accurate assessment and tailored treatment. Pain intensity scales and consistent monitoring guide the choice of analgesic therapies. Special attention should be given to pediatric patients, and opioids must be used judiciously to balance pain relief with potential adverse effects.

Anemia: A Comprehensive Overview

Anemia is defined as a condition in which hemoglobin (Hb) levels fall below the established reference values. These values vary based on factors such as age, gender, and pregnancy status (see Table 2 for reference).

Causes of Anaemia

Anemia can result from a range of interconnected causes, which include:

9

Decreased Red Blood Cell Production: This may occur due to iron deficiency, nutritional deficiencies (e.g., folic acid, vitamin B12, or vitamin A), impaired bone marrow function, certain infections (e.g., HIV, visceral leishmaniasis), or kidney failure.

Red Blood Cell Loss: Chronic or acute blood loss, such as from gastrointestinal ulcers or parasitic infections (e.g., ancylostomiasis, schistosomiasis), may lead to anemia.

Increased Red Blood Cell Destruction (Hemolysis): Conditions like malaria, bacterial or viral infections (e.g., HIV), and hemoglobinopathies (such as sickle cell disease or thalassemia) can cause premature red blood cell destruction. Additionally, drug-induced hemolysis can occur in individuals with G6PD deficiency (e.g., exposure to primaquine, dapsone, nitrofurantoin).

Clinical Features of Anaemia

Common symptoms include:

Pallor, especially of the conjunctiva, mucous membranes, palms, and soles.

Fatigue, dizziness, shortness of breath (dyspnoea), tachycardia, and heart murmurs.

Severe symptoms or signs of decompensation include:

Cold extremities, altered mental status, lower limb oedema, respiratory distress, elevated jugular venous pressure, and shock.

Additional specific signs may include:

Nutritional deficiencies (e.g., cheilosis and glossitis).
Jaundice, hepatosplenomegaly, and dark-colored urine (due to hemolysis).
Bleeding, such as melena or hematuria, may also be observed in some cases.

Diagnostic Workup

Full Blood Count (FBC): This provides an initial assessment, guiding the diagnostic process.
Microscopic Examination: Blood smears, including thick and thin films, should be examined, especially in malaria-endemic areas.
Urinary Dipstick Test: This can help detect hemoglobinuria or hematuria, which can point to hemolysis or bleeding.
Additional Tests: In cases of suspected sickle cell disease, rapid diagnostic tests such as Sickle SCAN® or Emmel test may be employed before administering blood transfusions.

Management

Anemia is not inherently an indication for blood transfusion, as many cases can be managed with etiological treatment alone. Blood transfusion is reserved for severe cases or when the clinical condition dictates.

Etiological Treatment: This often involves iron supplementation (ferrous salts) and folic acid. If iron deficiency or folate deficiency is the cause, these treatments are typically administered for a duration of 3-4 months.

Specific treatment recommendations based on anemia type include:

Iron Deficiency: Oral ferrous salts, with the appropriate dose for children and adults (e.g., 65 mg of elemental iron).

Folic Acid Deficiency: For children under 1 year, 0.5 mg/kg daily; for children 1 year and older and adults, 5 mg daily.

Classification of Anaemia Based on Red Blood Cell Size and Reticulocyte Count

Anemia can be classified as:

Macrocytic: Often caused by folic acid or vitamin B12 deficiencies, or chronic alcoholism.

Microcytic: Common in iron deficiency, thalassemia, or chronic inflammatory conditions (e.g., HIV infection, cancer).

Normocytic: Typically associated with acute hemorrhage, renal failure, or hemolysis.

The reticulocyte count further aids in classification:

Low Reticulocyte Count: Indicates a deficiency in production (e.g., iron, folic acid, or vitamin B12 deficiencies).

Normal or High Reticulocyte Count: Suggests increased red blood cell destruction (hemolysis), seen in conditions like sickle cell disease or thalassemia.

Blood Transfusion Considerations

When transfusion is indicated, the volume to be transfused should be based on the patient's clinical condition. For children, transfusion thresholds should be carefully monitored and adapted depending on symptoms like fever, ongoing blood loss, or severe infections.

Transfusion Volume for Children:

In the absence of fever, 15 ml/kg of packed red blood cells (PRBC) should be transfused over 3 hours.

If fever is present, 10 ml/kg of PRBC should be transfused over 3 hours.

Transfusion Volume for Adults and Adolescents: An adult unit of PRBC or whole blood should be administered, not exceeding 5 ml/kg/hour.

Monitoring During and After Transfusion

Patients undergoing blood transfusion should be closely monitored, with vital signs checked regularly (e.g., heart rate, blood pressure, temperature). Monitoring should include:

Every 5 minutes for the first 15 minutes, then every 30 minutes until transfusion is completed.

Post-transfusion checks should be done 4-6 hours after completion to detect any transfusion reactions or signs of fluid overload.

If circulatory overload is suspected, transfusion should be temporarily halted. The patient should be seated upright, oxygen administered, and furosemide given if required.

Prevention and Ongoing Management

Prevention of anemia involves addressing its underlying causes. This may include:
Iron and Folic Acid Supplementation: Especially in pregnancy, malnutrition, and other at-risk groups.
Management of Helminthic Infections: Conditions like schistosomiasis and nematode infections should be treated promptly.
Iron Deficiency Prevention Recommendations
Children 1 month to <12 years: 1-2 mg/kg daily, with a maximum dose of 65 mg/day.
Children ≥12 years and adults: 65 mg daily.
Anaemia Transfusion Thresholds
Children 2-6 months: Hb <9.5 g/dL indicates potential transfusion needs.
Children 6 months-4 years: Hb <11 g/dL warrants consideration for transfusion.
Adults: For men, Hb <13 g/dL, and for women, Hb <12 g/dL may be a trigger for transfusion if accompanied by decompensation or severe illness.

References

1. World Health Organization. Hemoglobin Concentrations for the Diagnosis of Anaemia and Assessment of Severity. World Health Organization; 2011.
2. World Health Organization. Educational Modules on Clinical Use of Blood. World Health Organization; 2021.
3. Maitland K, Olupot-Olupot P, Kiguli S, et al. Transfusion Volume for Children with Severe Anemia in Africa. N Engl J Med. 2019;381(5):420-431.
4. World Health Organization. Daily Iron and Folic Acid Supplementation in Pregnant Women. World Health Organization; 2012.

Dehydration Management and Treatment Protocols

Dehydration occurs when the body loses more water and electrolytes than it takes in. If left untreated, this can lead to reduced organ perfusion, potentially progressing to shock. Common causes include diarrhea, vomiting, and severe burns. Children are especially at risk due to frequent gastroenteritis episodes, their higher surface-area-to-volume ratio, and their inability to effectively communicate or independently manage fluid intake.

This guideline specifically addresses dehydration caused by diarrhea and vomiting. Separate protocols should be followed for children with malnutrition (refer to Chapter 1 on Severe Acute Malnutrition) or for those with severe burns (see Chapter 10 on Burns).

Clinical Features and Assessment
Classifying Dehydration Severity (adapted from WHO)

The degree of dehydration is assessed based on the following clinical features:

Severe Dehydration:
Lethargy or unconsciousness
Weak or absent radial pulse
Sunken eyes
Slow skin pinch (>2 seconds)
Inability to drink or very poor drinking ability

Some Dehydration:
Restlessness or irritability
Palpable radial pulse
Sunken eyes
Slow skin pinch (<2 seconds)
Thirsty, drinks quickly

No Dehydration:

Normal mental status
Easily palpable radial pulse
Normal eyes
Skin pinch returns quickly (<1 second)
Normal thirst and drinking behavior
Signs of Shock: In severe cases, dehydration can lead to shock, characterized by tachycardia, low blood pressure, and delayed capillary refill time. Additionally, electrolyte imbalances can cause symptoms such as tachypnoea, muscle cramps, weakness, arrhythmias, confusion, and seizures.
Treatment Protocols
Severe Dehydration: WHO Treatment Plan C
Immediate Action: Administer intravenous (IV) fluids for rapid rehydration. If the patient can drink, provide oral rehydration solution (ORS) while preparing for IV access.
IV Fluid Administration:
Children <1 year: Administer 30 ml/kg over 1 hour, followed by 70 ml/kg over 5 hours.
Children ≥1 year and adults: Administer 30 ml/kg over 30

minutes, followed by 70 ml/kg over 2.5 hours.
Repeat fluid bolus if the radial pulse remains weak or absent after initial administration.
Ringer's Lactate (RL) or 0.9% sodium chloride is used for rehydration. If severe anemia is suspected, a hemoglobin test should be conducted, and treatment should follow the guidelines in Chapter 1 on Anaemia.
Switching to Oral Rehydration: Once the patient is stable and able to drink, switch to ORS according to the patient's tolerance.
Ongoing Monitoring and Adjustments:
Electrolyte Imbalances: Monitor for signs of hypokalemia (muscle cramps/weakness, abdominal distention) and treat with potassium chloride syrup if needed.
Fluid Overload Signs: In cases of periorbital or peripheral oedema, slow the IV infusion rate and assess for complications such as respiratory distress (dyspnoea, cough, bibasal crepitations). Administer furosemide (1 mg/kg

in children; 40 mg in adults) if needed.

Dyspnoea or Pulmonary Edema: For patients showing signs of respiratory distress, reduce the IV infusion rate and administer furosemide, monitoring closely for improvement or worsening.

Some Dehydration: WHO Treatment Plan B

Oral Rehydration: Administer 75 ml/kg ORS over 4 hours, adjusting as necessary based on ongoing losses (e.g., loose stools).

Diarrhea Treatment in Children

In addition to the rehydration protocols, ensure that age-appropriate ORS volumes are administered:

Children <4 months: 200-400 ml over 4 hours

Children 4-11 months: 400-600 ml

Children 12-23 months: 600-800 ml

Children 2-4 years: 800-1200 ml

Children 5-14 years: 1200-2200 ml

Adults and children ≥15 years: 2200-4000 ml

Encourage additional age-appropriate fluid intake,

including breastfeeding for young children. After each episode of diarrhea, give additional ORS.

Aetiologic Treatment

If necessary, administer appropriate treatment for the underlying cause of diarrhea and provide zinc supplementation to children under 5 years to reduce the duration of the illness and prevent complications.

Conclusion

This protocol provides structured treatment strategies based on the degree of dehydration and specific clinical features. It emphasizes the importance of early intervention, close monitoring, and appropriate adjustments in therapy, particularly when complications such as shock or electrolyte imbalances arise.

References:

1. World Health Organization. The treatment of diarrhea: A manual for physicians and other senior health workers, 4th rev. World Health Organization. 2005.
2. World Health Organization. Pocket book of Hospital Care for

children. Guidelines for the Management of Common Childhood Illnesses. 2013.

Severe Acute Malnutrition (SAM) – Clinical Management and Protocols

Overview and Definitions

Severe acute malnutrition (SAM) arises from insufficient intake of essential nutrients, including energy (kilocalories), protein, fat, and micronutrients (vitamins and minerals), failing to meet the individual's nutritional requirements. SAM is often associated with significant medical complications due to metabolic disturbances, weakened immunity, and systemic effects. It remains a leading cause of morbidity and mortality, especially among children under five years of age.

This protocol focuses on the diagnosis and management of SAM in children aged 6 to 59 months. For other age groups, refer to national guidelines or specialized protocols.

Clinical Assessment of SAM

Physical Signs for Diagnosis:

Marasmus: Characterized by significant muscle wasting and

loss of subcutaneous fat, leading to a skeletal appearance.

Kwashiorkor: Typically presents with bilateral lower limb oedema, which can extend to other parts of the body (e.g., arms, face). Other signs include discolored, brittle hair, and shiny, cracked skin prone to infection.

Diagnostic Criteria: Diagnosis of SAM combines anthropometric measurements and clinical features:

Mid-Upper Arm Circumference (MUAC): A MUAC less than 115 mm indicates SAM and significant risk of mortality.

Weight-for-Height Z-score (WHZ): SAM is defined when WHZ is below -3 according to WHO Child Growth Standards.

Oedema: The presence of bilateral pitting oedema in the lower limbs, when other causes are excluded, confirms SAM, regardless of MUAC and WHZ.

Admission Criteria for SAM Treatment Programs: Admission protocols may vary by context and should align with local guidelines. Medical complications or severe symptoms (e.g., shock, seizures, severe dehydration) may require hospitalization.

Management of SAM

Initial Medical Management: Children with SAM often present with medical complications, necessitating careful management. Common issues include infections, dehydration, and anemia. They should be carefully monitored and treated with appropriate interventions such as:

1. Nutritional Treatment:

Phase 1 (Stabilization): Administer F-75 therapeutic milk for 1 to 7 days to stabilize metabolic functions and treat acute complications.

Transition Phase: Use F-100 therapeutic milk and/or ready-to-use therapeutic food (RUTF) to ensure continued improvement and tolerance of food intake.

Phase 2 (Catch-up Growth): Once stable, transition to RUTF for rapid weight gain and recovery. This phase may continue for several weeks with outpatient follow-up.

2. Breastfeeding: Continue breastfeeding in children who are

breastfed, as it provides essential nutrients and immunity.
3. Hydration and Electrolytes: Oral rehydration solutions (ORS) and ReSoMal may be used to prevent dehydration, especially in children with diarrhea. Monitor the child's hydration status regularly and adjust fluid intake as necessary.
Antibiotic Treatment: Routine antibiotics should be initiated on Day 1 for all children with SAM, unless specific infection signs are absent. A typical regimen includes:
Amoxicillin: 50 mg/kg orally twice daily for 5 to 7 days
Malaria: Rapid diagnostic tests and appropriate antimalarial treatment should be given if indicated, based on the results.
Intestinal Parasites: Albendazole administration as part of the transition phase to address intestinal helminths.
Vaccination:
Ensure children in the 6 to 59 months age group receive necessary vaccines, including measles and other EPI vaccines. If vaccines are delayed, re-vaccination should be planned

once the child reaches the appropriate age.

Managing Complications in SAM

1. Infections:

Respiratory, urinary, and cutaneous infections are common. In severe cases, sepsis may be suspected, particularly if the child is lethargic or in shock. Administer broad-spectrum antibiotics (e.g., ampicillin and gentamicin) and adjust based on the source of infection.

Children with kwashiorkor may have infected skin lesions. Transition antibiotics to amoxicillin/clavulanic acid for better skin infection control.

2. Severe Anemia:

Children with a hemoglobin level below 6 g/dl, or with signs of decompensated anemia, require urgent blood transfusion (preferably packed red blood cells).

3. Diarrhea and Dehydration:

SAM children are prone to dehydration, with signs such as lethargy and reduced urine output. Diarrhea should be treated with therapeutic foods and rehydration solutions.

Rehydration Protocols:
Plan A (no dehydration): Encourage breastfeeding and administer ORS as needed.
Plan B (some dehydration): Administer ReSoMal orally or via nasogastric tube (NGT) to address fluid loss.
Plan C (severe dehydration): If dehydration is severe, intravenous fluids such as G5%-RL should be given. If vomiting or severe fluid loss occurs, use IV rehydration and monitor closely for fluid overload.
4. Hypoglycaemia:
Monitor blood glucose levels regularly and treat hypoglycemia with appropriate glucose solutions as outlined in local protocols.
Outpatient Management
Children without severe medical complications may be managed as outpatients once they have entered Phase 2 and are stable. Regular follow-up visits are essential to monitor progress, address complications, and ensure continued nutritional recovery.
Key Steps:

Continue RUTF or therapeutic milk until the child achieves an adequate weight gain.
Provide ongoing vaccination and parasite control as needed.
Ensure the child is kept hydrated, and appropriate antibiotics are continued if needed.
Conclusion
SAM is a critical medical condition requiring prompt and structured intervention. Early diagnosis, tailored nutritional support, and management of medical complications are vital to improving outcomes. By following evidence-based protocols and ensuring comprehensive care, including infection control, rehydration, and gradual nutritional rehabilitation, healthcare providers can significantly reduce the morbidity and mortality associated with SAM.

Chapter 2
Respiratory Diseases
This chapter reviews various respiratory conditions, their pathophysiology, and the importance of early recognition and intervention to prevent

complications and improve patient outcomes:

Acute Upper Airway Obstruction: Explores the causes and clinical signs of upper airway blockage, emphasizing the critical need for rapid intervention to prevent respiratory failure and ensure airway patency.

Rhinitis and Rhinopharyngitis (Common Cold): Discusses the viral origin of these conditions, symptoms like congestion and sore throat, and the importance of symptomatic treatment to manage discomfort and prevent secondary infections.

Acute Sinusitis: Reviews the inflammatory process in the sinuses, often following a cold, and the need for appropriate treatment to alleviate symptoms and prevent chronic or recurrent sinus infections.

Acute Pharyngitis: Focuses on the causes of sore throat, including viral and bacterial pathogens, and highlights the importance of differentiating bacterial infections like streptococcal pharyngitis for targeted therapy.

Diphtheria: Examines this potentially life-threatening bacterial infection, stressing the urgency of early diagnosis and the administration of antitoxin and antibiotics to prevent airway obstruction and systemic complications.

Other Upper Respiratory Tract Infections: Reviews a range of infections affecting the upper respiratory system, underscoring the importance of early identification and supportive care in preventing more severe conditions.

Croup (Laryngotracheitis and Laryngotracheobronchitis): Discusses the viral etiology of croup, its hallmark barking cough, and the need for supportive treatments such as corticosteroids and nebulized epinephrine to reduce airway swelling.

Epiglottitis: Reviews the life-threatening bacterial infection of the epiglottis, its rapid progression, and the need for emergent airway management to prevent suffocation.

Bacterial Tracheitis: Focuses on the severe bacterial infection of the trachea, stressing the importance of timely antibiotics and airway support to prevent respiratory failure.

Otitis: Reviews various ear infections, including acute otitis and otitis media, emphasizing the need for antibiotics in bacterial cases and addressing potential complications like hearing loss.

Acute Otitis Externa: Discusses the common bacterial or fungal causes of outer ear infections and the role of topical treatment to manage symptoms.

Acute Otitis Media (AOM): Explains the middle ear infection in children, often caused by bacteria, and the need for antibiotics in bacterial cases to prevent complications.

Chronic Suppurative Otitis Media (CSOM): Reviews the persistent middle ear infection that can lead to long-term hearing impairment and the need for appropriate medical or surgical management.

Whooping Cough (Pertussis): Discusses this highly contagious bacterial infection, its symptoms, and the critical need for early antibiotic treatment and vaccination to prevent complications, especially in infants.

Bronchitis: Reviews both acute and chronic forms of bronchitis, highlighting the viral causes of acute bronchitis and the long-term management of chronic bronchitis to reduce symptoms and prevent exacerbations.

Acute Bronchitis: Focuses on the viral etiology of acute bronchitis and the supportive care needed to manage cough and inflammation.

Chronic Bronchitis: Discusses the long-term condition, often due to smoking, that requires ongoing management to control symptoms and improve quality of life.

Bronchiolitis: Explores the viral infection of small airways, particularly in infants, and stresses the importance of supportive care and close monitoring to prevent respiratory distress.

Acute Pneumonia: Reviews the pathophysiology of pneumonia, including the common bacterial and viral causes, and emphasizes the need for timely antibiotic treatment and supportive care to prevent complications.

Pneumonia in Children Under 5 Years: Discusses the unique risks for young children and the importance of early diagnosis and treatment to prevent severe outcomes.

Pneumonia in Children Over 5 Years and Adults: Reviews the common causes of pneumonia in older children and adults, with an emphasis on bacterial pathogens and appropriate treatment strategies.

Persistent Pneumonia: Discusses the management of pneumonia that does not resolve with standard treatment, often indicating resistant pathogens or complications that require specialized care.

Staphylococcal Pneumonia: Focuses on the severe form of pneumonia caused by Staphylococcus species, requiring aggressive antibiotic therapy to manage.

Asthma: Reviews the chronic inflammatory disease of the airways, emphasizing the importance of both acute and long-term management to control symptoms and prevent exacerbations.

Acute Asthma Attack: Discusses the triggers and management of acute asthma exacerbations, focusing on bronchodilators and corticosteroids to relieve symptoms.

Chronic Asthma: Highlights the need for long-term medication and lifestyle management to prevent asthma attacks and improve quality of life.

Pulmonary Tuberculosis: Reviews this serious bacterial infection of the lungs, emphasizing the importance of prolonged antibiotic therapy and early diagnosis to prevent spread and complications.

Acute Upper Airway Obstruction: Management and Approach

Acute upper airway obstruction can arise from various causes, including foreign body aspiration, viral and bacterial infections (such as croup, epiglottitis, and tracheitis), anaphylaxis, burns, or trauma. Initially, an obstruction may appear stable, but it can rapidly progress into a life-threatening situation, especially in young children.

Clinical Features

The severity of the obstruction can be identified through various clinical signs:

1. Complete Obstruction

Danger Signs: Respiratory distress progressing to cardiac arrest, severe respiratory distress with cyanosis or $SpO2 < 90\%$, agitation or lethargy, tachycardia, capillary refill > 3 seconds, severe stridor, and severe retractions.

Management: Immediate intervention is required, with continuous monitoring of SpO2, heart rate, respiratory rate, and mental status. Administer oxygen to maintain SpO2 between 94-98%. If SpO2 monitoring is unavailable, administer oxygen at 5 L/min or more to relieve hypoxia.

2. Severe Respiratory Distress

Signs: Severe intercostal, subcostal, and substernal retractions, nasal flaring, severe tachypnoea.

Management: Supportive care with oxygen therapy, monitoring vitals, and close observation for signs of deterioration. Hospitalization is necessary, potentially in an intensive care setting if danger signs are present.

3. Moderate Obstruction

Signs: Moderate stridor with agitation, mild intercostal and subcostal retractions, moderate tachypnoea.

Management: Continue monitoring and oxygen administration. Hospitalization may be required depending on progression.

4. Mild Obstruction

Signs: Mild cough, hoarseness, no respiratory distress.

Management: Observation, supportive care, and monitoring SpO2 if needed. Most cases do not require hospitalization.

General Management:

Position the child or adult in a comfortable position to ease breathing.

For severe cases, administer oxygen to maintain SpO2 between 94-98%.

In cases of mild obstruction, continuous monitoring is sufficient, with hydration management if necessary (oral or IV).

Management of Foreign Body Aspiration

Foreign body aspiration can result in acute airway obstruction, commonly occurring in children aged 6 months to 5 years while playing with small objects or eating. In these cases, the child may initially remain conscious.

Intervention Guidelines:

For an adult or child unable to cough, speak, or make any sound:

Heimlich Maneuver: Stand behind the patient, place a closed fist above the navel, and apply quick, upward thrusts to expel the foreign body.

For infants: Place the infant face down across your forearm, supporting their head, and administer five back slaps. If unsuccessful, turn the infant onto their back and perform five sternal compressions.

If unsuccessful and the patient loses consciousness, initiate ventilation and CPR. A tracheostomy may be required if ventilation fails.

Management of Airway Obstruction due to Infections

Infections are a common cause of airway obstruction, particularly in children. The presentation and management vary based on the causative pathogen:

1. Viral Croup (Children over 1 year)

Symptoms: Stridor, cough, moderate respiratory distress.

Management: Usually resolves with supportive care, corticosteroids, and nebulized epinephrine to reduce airway inflammation.

2. Epiglottitis (Children and Adults)

Symptoms: High fever, stridor, severe respiratory distress, drooling, difficulty swallowing.

Management: Emergency management is required with intubation if necessary, and intravenous antibiotics to treat the bacterial infection.

3. Bacterial Tracheitis (Children)

Symptoms: Fever, purulent secretions, severe respiratory distress, stridor.

Management: IV antibiotics, often requiring mechanical ventilation for airway support.

4. Retropharyngeal or Tonsillar Abscess (Children)

Symptoms: Fever, sore throat, painful swallowing, earache, trismus, hot potato voice.

Management: Surgical drainage is typically required to resolve the abscess.

Management for Burns or Smoke Inhalation:

Burns to the face or neck and smoke inhalation can cause airway edema and obstruction, requiring immediate intervention with airway management and oxygen supplementation.

Anaphylactic Reaction:

In cases of anaphylaxis with airway involvement (angioedema), rapid administration of epinephrine and airway support is crucial, as outlined in the management of anaphylactic shock (Chapter 1).

Conclusion:

Effective management of acute upper airway obstruction requires early recognition of symptoms, appropriate interventions based on the severity of obstruction, and constant monitoring to prevent progression to life-threatening conditions.

Footnote
(a) Whenever possible, it is recommended to administer oxygen to all patients with an SpO2 level below 95%.

Rhinitis and Rhinopharyngitis (Common Cold)

Rhinitis, characterized by inflammation of the nasal mucosa, and rhinopharyngitis, involving both the nasal and pharyngeal mucosa, are typically mild and self-limited conditions, most commonly caused by viral infections. However, these conditions can sometimes be the initial symptoms of more serious illnesses, such as measles or influenza, or may lead to secondary bacterial infections, including otitis media or sinusitis.

Clinical Features

Common symptoms include nasal discharge or blockage, sore throat, fever, cough, lacrimation (tearing), and in infants, diarrhea. It is important to note that purulent (thick, yellow or green) nasal discharge does not necessarily indicate a secondary bacterial infection.

For children under the age of 5, it is recommended to regularly check the tympanic membranes for signs of otitis media, which can often accompany rhinitis or rhinopharyngitis.

Treatment

Antibiotic therapy is generally not indicated, as it does not expedite recovery or reduce the risk of complications.

Management is symptomatic, focusing on alleviating discomfort:

Nasal Congestion: Use 0.9% sodium chloride solution to help clear the nasal passages.

Fever and Sore Throat: Administer paracetamol orally for 2 to 3 days as needed to reduce fever and alleviate throat pain.

Footnote

(a) For infants, position the child on their back with the head turned to the side, then gently instill 0.9% sodium chloride solution into each nostril to clear the nasal passages.

Acute Sinusitis

Acute sinusitis refers to the inflammation of one or more sinus cavities, commonly caused by either an infection or allergic reaction. Most cases are viral and tend to resolve without intervention within 10 days, with treatment focused on symptom management. However, bacterial sinusitis can arise as a primary infection, a complication of viral sinusitis, or as a result of a dental infection. The primary bacterial culprits include Streptococcus pneumoniae, Haemophilus influenzae, and Moraxella . Distinguishing bacterial sinusitis from common viral rhinitis is essential for proper management. Antibiotics are only necessary for bacterial infections.

If left untreated, severe sinusitis in children can lead to complications such as the spread of infection to adjacent bony structures, the orbit, or even the meninges.

Clinical Features

Sinusitis in Adults

Sinusitis is suspected if symptoms persist for more than 10-14 days, worsen after 5-7 days, or are severe (e.g., intense pain, high fever, or general deterioration in health).

Sinusitis in Children

In addition to the usual symptoms (nasal discharge, obstruction, facial pain), children may exhibit irritability, lethargy, cough, or vomiting. Severe infections can lead to deterioration in the child's condition, with high fever (>39°C) and periorbital or facial swelling.

Treatment

Symptomatic Treatment

For nasal congestion, clear the nose using 0.9% sodium chloride solution (see footnote).

Fever and pain can be managed with paracetamol (refer to Chapter 1 on Fever).

Antibiotherapy

Adults

Antibiotics are indicated when symptoms persist beyond the expected duration or are of significant severity. Oral amoxicillin is the first-line treatment. If the diagnosis is unclear or symptoms are moderate and less than 10 days in duration, symptomatic treatment for viral sinusitis or rhinitis may be sufficient.

Children

Antibiotics are recommended for children with severe symptoms or mild symptoms with risk factors such as immunosuppression, asthma, or sickle cell disease. The first-line antibiotic for children is oral amoxicillin, dosed as follows:
Children: 30 mg/kg three times daily (maximum 3g daily)
Adults: 1g three times daily
If no improvement is observed within 48 hours, switch to amoxicillin/clavulanic acid for 7-10 days. For children under 40 kg, the dose is 25 mg/kg twice daily, while children and adults above 40 kg should receive 2000 mg daily (8:1 ratio) or 1750 mg daily (7:1 ratio).
For patients allergic to penicillin, erythromycin is an alternative, dosed as:
Children: 30 to 50 mg/kg daily
Adults: 1g two to three times daily
In cases of sinusitis secondary to dental infections, dental extraction may be necessary in conjunction with ongoing antibiotic therapy. For complications involving the eye (e.g., ophthalmoplegia, reduced

vision), refer for surgical drainage.

Footnotes

(a) For infants, place the child on their back with the head turned to the side and instill 0.9% sodium chloride into each nostril to clear the nose.

(b) For specific erythromycin doses, refer to the Essential Drugs guide.

Acute Pharyngitis: A Detailed Overview

Introduction

Acute pharyngitis refers to the inflammation of the tonsils and pharynx, which is most commonly caused by viral infections. While most cases resolve without antibiotics, Group A Streptococcus (GAS) is a key bacterial pathogen, especially in children aged 3 to 14 years. Early identification of the cause is critical, as appropriate antibiotic treatment for GAS can prevent complications such as Acute Rheumatic Fever (ARF).

Clinical Features

Pharyngitis presents with symptoms like sore throat, difficulty swallowing, inflamed tonsils, and tender anterior cervical lymph nodes, with or without fever. The appearance of the throat can range from erythematous (redness) to exudative (presence of white spots), which is common in both viral and GAS infections.

Viral Pharyngitis: Commonly caused by viruses such as Epstein-Barr virus (EBV) or Coxsackievirus. In cases of infectious mononucleosis (IM), the presence of extreme fatigue, generalized adenopathy, and splenomegaly is typical.

Bacterial Pharyngitis: GAS infections in children often present with erythematous or exudative pharyngitis. The Centor criteria are useful for distinguishing bacteria from viral causes and minimizing unnecessary antibiotic prescriptions when rapid testing for GAS is unavailable.

Centor Criteria for GAS Pharyngitis

The Centor score helps assess the likelihood of GAS infection. A score of 0-1 suggests a viral cause, while scores ≥ 2 indicate

the need for antibiotic treatment. The criteria include:
1. Temperature >38°C: 1 point
2. Absence of cough: 1 point
3. Tender anterior cervical lymph node(s): 1 point
4. Tonsillar swelling or exudate: 1 point

A score of 0-1 typically suggests viral pharyngitis, which does not require antibiotics. A higher score, or the presence of scarlet fever, warrants treatment for GAS.

Differential Diagnosis

Other causes of pharyngitis include:

Gonococcal or HIV pharyngitis: Associated with specific risk factors and patient history.

Diphtheria: Characterized by pseudomembranous pharyngitis, presenting as a grayish-white membrane.

Herpetic or Vesicular Pharyngitis: Caused by viruses like Coxsackievirus or primary herpes simplex virus infection, marked by small blisters or ulcers on the tonsils.

Peritonsillar, Retropharyngeal, or Lateral Pharyngeal Abscesses: Present with severe symptoms such as fever, intense pain, difficulty swallowing, hoarseness, and trismus.

Treatment

Treatment of acute pharyngitis depends on the underlying cause:

1. Symptomatic Treatment: For viral pharyngitis or mild bacterial cases (Centor score <2), symptomatic management with analgesics like paracetamol or ibuprofen is recommended.

2. Antibiotic Therapy for GAS Pharyngitis:

First-line: Benzathine benzylpenicillin (IM) is the treatment of choice. It has proven efficacy in preventing ARF.

Children (<30 kg): 600,000 IU (single dose)

Children ≥30 kg, Adults: 1.2 million IU (single dose)

Oral Penicillin V can also be used but may lead to poor adherence due to its longer treatment course.

Children 1-6 years: 250 mg twice daily

Children 6-12 years: 500 mg twice daily

Children ≥12 years and adults: 1 g twice daily

Alternative: Amoxicillin for 6 days (particularly for children) with a dosage of 25 mg/kg twice daily, or 1 g twice daily for adults.

Macrolides: Used for patients allergic to penicillin. Azithromycin for 3 days (adults: 500 mg once daily, children: 20 mg/kg once daily) is effective but should be reserved due to resistance concerns.

3. Other Considerations:

Gonococcal or Syphilitic Pharyngitis: Treatment follows guidelines for gonorrhea and syphilis.

Diphtheria Pharyngitis: Managed as described under the Diphtheria section.

Vincent's Tonsillitis: Treated with metronidazole or amoxicillin.

Abscess Formation: In the case of peritonsillar, retropharyngeal, or lateral pharyngeal abscesses, surgical drainage may be necessary.

Complications and Follow-Up

For severe cases, such as those presenting with symptoms of ARF, acute glomerulonephritis, or epiglottitis, early hospitalization and intensive treatment are necessary. Signs of serious illness in children include severe dehydration, difficulty swallowing, and respiratory distress, which require urgent medical intervention.

Conclusion

Acute pharyngitis is most commonly viral but can be caused by bacterial infections like GAS, which require targeted antibiotic therapy. Identifying the cause through clinical assessment, such as using the Centor criteria, is crucial for effective management. Antibiotic treatment should be reserved for bacterial infections, especially to prevent complications such as ARF. Prompt diagnosis and appropriate treatment can significantly reduce morbidity and prevent complications.

References

1. Fine AM, Nizet V, Mandl KD. Large-scale validation of the Centor and McIsaac scores to predict group A streptococcal pharyngitis. Arch Intern Med. 2012;172(11):847-852.
2. National Institute for Health and Care Excellence. Sore throat

(acute): antimicrobial prescribing. 2018.
3. Centers for Disease Control and Prevention. Group A Streptococcal Disease, 2020.

Diphtheria: A Comprehensive Overview

Last Updated: October 2022

Diphtheria is a serious bacterial infection caused by Corynebacterium . It primarily spreads through respiratory droplets from infected individuals, who may either be symptomatic or asymptomatic, or by direct contact with contaminated surfaces or skin lesions. The incubation period for C. diphtheriae typically ranges from 1 to 5 days, with a maximum of 10 days, during which the bacteria multiply in the upper respiratory tract. The bacteria secrete a potent toxin that causes severe localized and systemic effects. The complications of diphtheria include airway obstruction and systemic effects such as myocarditis and nerve damage, which can result in death if not treated promptly. Patients may remain infectious for up to 8 weeks, although antibiotic treatment can shorten this period to 6 days.

Prevention and Vaccination

Vaccination is the cornerstone of diphtheria prevention. The vaccine reduces the severity of symptoms but does not entirely prevent the spread of the bacteria. Infected individuals do not acquire immunity from the disease itself, underscoring the importance of vaccination in preventing future cases. Vaccination is crucial in the management of diphtheria, as clinical disease does not confer protective immunity.

Clinical Features

The clinical presentation of respiratory diphtheria often involves sore throat (pharyngitis), nasal congestion (rhinopharyngitis), tonsillitis, or laryngitis, accompanied by tough, grayish pseudomembranes in the affected areas such as the pharynx, nasopharynx, tonsils, or larynx. Other signs include dysphagia (difficulty swallowing) and cervical adenitis, which may progress to significant neck swelling. As the

infection progresses, it can obstruct the airway, leading to suffocation, especially when it extends to the nasal passages, larynx, trachea, and bronchi. Fever is typically low-grade.
Toxin-related complications can be systemic and include cardiac dysfunction such as tachycardia, arrhythmias, and severe myocarditis, which may lead to heart failure and cardiogenic shock 3 to 7 days after disease onset. Neuropathy can develop 2 to 8 weeks post-infection, resulting in symptoms such as nasal speech, difficulty swallowing (due to soft palate paralysis), vision issues (ocular motor paralysis), respiratory issues (paralysis of respiratory muscles), and limb paralysis. In some cases, acute renal failure can occur, with symptoms like oliguria or anuria.

Differential Diagnosis

Diphtheria should be differentiated from conditions such as epiglottitis, acute pharyngitis, and stomatitis, which present with similar symptoms.

Diagnosis

Diagnosis is confirmed by culturing a sample from the affected area (e.g., throat, tonsils, or nasopharynx) and performing an antibiotic susceptibility test. PCR testing can detect the diphtheria toxin gene, confirming the presence of the toxin. Early isolation of the patient and implementation of standard, droplet, and contact precautions are essential to prevent the spread of the infection.

Treatment

Immediate treatment is critical and should not be delayed while awaiting bacteriological confirmation. Diphtheria antitoxin (DAT), derived from horse serum, should be administered as soon as the diagnosis is suspected. The Besredka method is used to assess possible allergic reactions to antitoxin. Delays in administering the antitoxin can reduce its effectiveness. Doses vary depending on the severity of the disease and the time elapsed since symptom onset.

In patients with penicillin allergy, alternatives such as erythromycin or azithromycin should be used. Antibiotic treatment is typically continued for 14 days, with appropriate dosing based on the patient's age and weight.

Management of Close Contacts

Close contacts, including household members and individuals who have been in close proximity to the patient (less than 1 meter) for a prolonged period, should receive prophylactic antibiotic treatment, even in the absence of symptoms. This includes benzathine benzylpenicillin or azithromycin/erythromycin for a duration of 7 days. Additionally, the vaccination status of close contacts should be reviewed and updated if necessary.

Outbreak Surveillance and Prevention

In the event of an outbreak, public health measures include routine vaccination with a conjugate diphtheria vaccine, which is typically administered in a three-dose series starting at 6 weeks of age, followed by boosters at 12-23 months and again at 4-7 years. A booster dose should be administered to individuals over 7 years of age, particularly during outbreaks. Individuals who are unvaccinated or incompletely vaccinated should undergo catch-up vaccination. Regular surveillance, including nasal and throat swabs, should be conducted during outbreaks to monitor for new cases.

Vaccination Schedule

For children, routine vaccination includes 3 doses of the conjugate diphtheria toxoid vaccine, with a booster at 12-23 months, followed by another booster at 4-7 years. Adolescents and adults who are at risk of exposure, including healthcare workers, should also receive booster doses as necessary. During outbreaks, vaccination intervals may be shortened to ensure rapid immunity.

Conclusion

Diphtheria remains a preventable yet potentially fatal disease, emphasizing the need for vigilant vaccination programs, early detection, and prompt treatment. Although the disease has become rare in many countries due to widespread vaccination, it still poses a significant threat in regions with lower vaccination coverage. Comprehensive case management, including timely administration of antitoxin and antibiotics, is crucial in reducing mortality and preventing transmission.

References

1. World Health Organization. Diphtheria: Vaccine-Preventable Diseases Surveillance Standards. 2018.
2. Tiwari TSP, Wharton M. Diphtheria Toxoid. In: Plotkin SA, Orenstein WA, Ofit PA, editors. Vaccines. 7th ed. Philadelphia, PA: Elsevier; 2018.
3. Truelove SA, Keegan LT, Moss WJ, et al. Clinical and Epidemiological Aspects of Diphtheria: A Systematic Review and Pooled Analysis. Clin Infect Dis. 2020.
4. Pan American Health Organization, World Health Organization. Diphtheria in the Americas: Summary of the Situation 2018. Epidemiological Update.
5. World Health Organization. Diphtheria Vaccine: WHO Position Paper - August 2017.

Weekly Epidemiological Record, 2017.
Other Upper Respiratory Tract Infections

1. Laryngotracheitis and Laryngotracheobronchitis (Croup)

Croup is an upper respiratory infection primarily affecting children, causing inflammation of the larynx, trachea, and bronchi. It is typically caused by viral agents, particularly parainfluenza viruses, and presents with symptoms such as a distinctive "barking" cough, hoarseness, and stridor (a high-pitched wheezing sound during breathing). The inflammation leads to narrowing of the airways, which can cause significant breathing difficulty, especially during the night. Management usually includes supportive care, humidified air, and corticosteroids to reduce airway inflammation. In severe cases, nebulized epinephrine or hospitalization may be required for respiratory distress.

2. Epiglottitis

Epiglottitis is a potentially life-threatening condition where the epiglottis, the cartilage that covers the windpipe, becomes inflamed and swollen, obstructing the airway. It is most often caused by Haemophilus influenzae type b (Hib) in unvaccinated children, though other bacteria like Streptococcus and Staphylococcus can also be responsible. The condition presents with rapid onset of severe sore throat, difficulty swallowing, drooling, and stridor. Epiglottitis requires urgent medical attention, often necessitating airway management through intubation or a tracheostomy to prevent suffocation. Antibiotic therapy is crucial to treat the underlying infection.

3. Bacterial Tracheitis

Bacterial tracheitis involves inflammation of the trachea, often as a result of bacterial infection following a viral upper respiratory infection. It is most commonly caused by Staphylococcus aureus, including methicillin-resistant Staphylococcus aureus (MRSA), and can cause symptoms similar to croup, including a cough, stridor, and respiratory distress. However, bacterial tracheitis typically presents with higher fever and more pronounced illness. Treatment usually includes intravenous antibiotics, and in some cases, mechanical ventilation may be required due to the severity of airway obstruction.

Croup (Laryngotracheitis and Laryngotracheobronchitis)

Last Updated: October 2024

Croup is a common viral respiratory infection, primarily affecting children between 6 months and 3 years of age. It involves inflammation of the larynx, trachea, and bronchi, which can lead to airway obstruction. The condition typically presents with a characteristic "barking" cough and inspiratory stridor (a high-pitched wheezing sound during inhalation), which can vary in severity.

Clinical Features:

Barking Cough: The hallmark symptom of croup, characterized by a harsh, seal-like cough.

Hoarse Voice or Cry: Due to inflammation of the vocal cords.

Inspiratory Stridor: Stridor that occurs only with agitation suggests mild croup, while stridor at rest, especially with respiratory distress, indicates severe croup.

Wheezing: May occur if the bronchi are involved, indicating more extensive airway inflammation.

Treatment:

Management of croup is based on the severity of the symptoms. In mild cases, where stridor is only present with agitation, treatment is primarily supportive.

1. Mild Croup (Stridor with Agitation):

Hydration: Ensure adequate fluid intake to prevent dehydration.

Corticosteroids:

Dexamethasone: 0.15 to 0.6 mg/kg (max. 16 mg) as a single dose.

Alternatively, Prednisolone: 1 mg/kg as a single dose.

Observation: Keep the child under observation for at least 30 minutes after administering corticosteroids. Extended observation (more than 4 hours) may be necessary for children under 6 months, those with dehydration, or those living far from a healthcare facility.

2. Severe Croup (Stridor at Rest or Respiratory Distress):

Oxygen: Administer continuous oxygen if respiratory distress or oxygen saturation (SpO2) drops below 92%. Target an SpO2 of 94-98% or, if SpO2 monitoring is unavailable, provide at least 5 liters/min of oxygen.

IV Hydration: Start an intravenous line to provide fluids if oral intake is not possible.

Nebulized Epinephrine: Administer 0.5 mg/kg (maximum 5 mg), repeated every 20 minutes if symptoms persist. This treatment helps to reduce airway swelling and improve breathing.

Note: Nebulized epinephrine should not be given intravenously or intramuscularly. During nebulization, monitor the child's heart rate, and stop the treatment if the heart rate exceeds 200 beats per minute.

3. In Case of Complications:

Hospitalization: Consider hospitalization if the child has persistent danger signs, such as severe stridor at rest, respiratory distress, or difficulty drinking.

Bacterial Tracheitis: In critically ill children with croup who do not improve with standard treatment, bacterial tracheitis should be suspected. This requires more aggressive management, including possible intubation or tracheostomy in the event of airway obstruction.

Dosing for Corticosteroids (Dexamethasone or Prednisolone):

Weight (kg)	Dexamethasone dose (mg)	Prednisolone dose (mg)
6 - 8 kg	4mg	6mg
6 - 11 kg	6mg	9mg
12 - 14 kg	8mg	12mg

Special Considerations:
Children with moderate to severe croup should be closely monitored for signs of airway compromise. Severe distress, difficulty in maintaining hydration, or inability to drink may warrant hospitalization.

Bacterial Tracheitis: In children with croup who do not improve with standard treatments, bacterial tracheitis should be considered. This condition is

characterized by the persistence of symptoms despite initial treatment with corticosteroids and nebulized epinephrine.
References
1. WHO Regional Office for Europe. Pocket book of primary health care for children and adolescents: guidelines for health promotion, disease prevention and management from the newborn period to adolescence. 2022.
2. Bjornson C, Russell K, Vandermeer B, Klassen TP, Johnson DW. Nebulized epinephrine for croup in children. Cochrane Database Syst Rev. Published online October 10, 2013.

Epiglottitis

Epiglottitis is a severe bacterial infection of the epiglottis, primarily affecting young children. It is commonly caused by Haemophilus influenzae type b (Hib), although it can also result from other bacteria. The incidence of Hib-related epiglottitis has significantly decreased in regions with high Hib vaccination coverage. This condition can also occur in adults.

Clinical Features

Rapid Onset: Symptoms usually develop quickly, within 12 to 24 hours, including high fever.

Tripod Position: Children often adopt the "tripod" or "sniffing" posture—sitting upright, leaning forward with an open mouth, and appearing anxious.

Swallowing Difficulties: Drooling and difficulty swallowing are common due to airway obstruction.

Stridor: Unlike croup, epiglottitis is characterized by inspiratory stridor (a high-pitched sound when breathing in), without hoarseness or a cough.

Respiratory Distress: The child may show signs of significant respiratory distress, and may appear critically ill. Signs of a critically ill child include weak or labored crying, drowsiness, difficulty arousing, lack of expression, pallor, or cyanosis.

Management

Positioning: Allow the child to sit comfortably or be held by a parent. Avoid forcing the child to lie down as this can worsen airway obstruction. Refrain from examining the throat as it may agitate the child and worsen symptoms.

Airway Management: If airway obstruction is imminent, immediate intervention is necessary. Intubation should be performed under general anesthesia by an experienced physician. If intubation is unsuccessful, tracheotomy may be required.

Treatment

1. IV Hydration: Establish a peripheral intravenous (IV) line and provide fluids to maintain hydration.

2. Antibiotic Therapy:

Ceftriaxone: Administer ceftriaxone via slow IV infusion or IV bolus (over 3-30 minutes). Avoid intramuscular (IM) injections, as they can cause agitation and trigger respiratory arrest.

For children: 50 mg/kg once daily.

For adults: 1 g once daily.

Continue IV treatment for at least 5 days, or until the patient's condition improves.

3. Switch to Oral Antibiotics: Once the child's condition has stabilized and they are able to tolerate oral medications, transition to oral antibiotics to complete a 7-10 day treatment course:

Amoxicillin/Clavulanic Acid (Co-Amoxiclav): This combination should be used exclusively in a ratio of either 8:1 or 7:1.

For children under 40 kg: 50 mg/kg, administered twice daily.

For children over 40 kg and adults:

8:1 ratio: 3000 mg daily (equivalent to two 500/62.5 mg tablets three times a day).

7:1 ratio: 2625 mg daily (equivalent to one 875/125 mg tablet three times a day).

Footnotes

Critically Ill Child: Signs of a critically ill child include weak crying, drowsiness, difficulty being aroused, lack of expression, pallor, or cyanosis.

Ceftriaxone Administration: When administering ceftriaxone IV, reconstitute it with water for injection. For infusion, dilute it with saline or glucose based on the child's weight and age.

Improvement Indicators: Improvement is indicated by fever reduction, reduced respiratory distress, improved oxygen saturation (SpO_2), and a better appetite and activity level.

Bacterial Tracheitis

Bacterial tracheitis is a serious infection of the trachea, often occurring as a secondary complication following a viral infection, such as croup, influenza, or measles. This condition is most commonly seen in children.

Clinical Features

Fever and Respiratory Distress: The child may appear critically ill, often with high fever, stridor, and a cough.

Purulent Secretions: The child may produce copious amounts of purulent (pus-like) secretions.

Gradual Onset: Unlike epiglottitis, bacterial tracheitis typically has a more gradual onset of symptoms. The child may prefer to lie flat, in contrast to the tripod position seen in epiglottitis.

Risk of Airway Obstruction: In severe cases, especially in very young children, there is a risk of complete airway obstruction, which requires immediate intervention.

Treatment

1. Airway Management:
Suctioning: Clear the trachea by suctioning purulent secretions to prevent airway blockage.
Intubation or Tracheostomy: In the event of complete airway obstruction, intubation should be attempted. If unsuccessful, an emergency tracheotomy may be necessary.
2. IV Hydration: Establish a peripheral IV line to administer fluids for hydration.
3. Antibiotic Therapy:
Ceftriaxone: Administer ceftriaxone via slow IV infusion or bolus (over 3-30 minutes). Avoid the intramuscular (IM) route, as it can agitate the child and lead to respiratory arrest.
For children: 50 mg/kg once daily.
For adults: 1 g once daily.
Cloxacillin: Administer IV cloxacillin over 60 minutes.

For children under 12 years: 25-50 mg/kg every 6 hours.
For children over 12 years and adults: 2 g every 6 hours.
4. Transition to Oral Antibiotics: After 5 days of IV antibiotics, if the child's condition has improved and they can tolerate oral medications, switch to amoxicillin/clavulanic acid (co-amoxiclav) for a total treatment duration of 7 to 10 days.

Footnotes

Critically Ill Child: Signs of a critically ill child include weak or labored crying, drowsiness, difficulty being aroused, lack of expression, pallor, cyanosis, or generalized hypotonia.

Ceftriaxone Administration: When administering ceftriaxone IV, it should be reconstituted with water for injection. For IV infusion, dilute with 0.9% sodium chloride or 5% glucose based on the child's weight.

Improvement Indicators: Clinical improvement can be assessed by a reduction in fever, decreased respiratory distress, improved oxygen saturation (SpO_2), and an increase in appetite or activity.

Otitis

Acute Otitis Externa (AOE)
Acute otitis , commonly known as swimmer's ear, is an infection of the outer ear canal. It is typically caused by bacterial infections, often due to water exposure, trauma to the ear canal, or skin conditions. Symptoms include itching, pain, swelling, and possible discharge from the ear. Treatment involves ear drops containing antibiotics and steroids, with attention to keeping the ear dry.

Acute Otitis Media (AOM)
Acute otitis media is an infection of the middle ear, frequently occurring after a cold, upper respiratory infection, or allergies. It is common in children. The condition is characterized by ear pain, fever, hearing loss, and irritability. The middle ear may be filled with fluid and pus, which can cause a bulging eardrum. Antibiotics may be prescribed for bacterial infections, though many cases resolve on their own.

Chronic Suppurative Otitis Media (CSOM)
Chronic suppurative otitis media is a long-lasting ear infection that

leads to persistent ear drainage (otorrhea) through a perforated eardrum. This condition is typically caused by bacterial infections that have not resolved properly or by complications from acute otitis media. CSOM may result in hearing loss, and the treatment usually involves prolonged antibiotic therapy and, in some cases, surgical intervention to repair the perforated eardrum and remove infected tissue.

Acute Otitis Externa

Acute otitis is characterized by inflammation of the external ear canal, typically caused by bacterial or fungal infections. Key risk factors include moisture exposure (maceration), trauma to the ear canal, foreign body presence, and dermatologic conditions like eczema or psoriasis.

Clinical Features

Ear symptoms: The condition presents with ear itching or pain, which is often severe and aggravated by pinna movement. A sensation of fullness in the ear is common. Discharge may be clear or purulent, or there may be no discharge at all.

Otoscopy: Upon examination, signs include diffuse redness and swelling of the ear canal, or infected eczema. A foreign body may be visible. The tympanic membrane usually appears normal, though its full assessment may be hindered due to swelling and pain in the ear canal.

Treatment

Pain Management: For pain relief, oral paracetamol can be used, as outlined in Chapter 1, Pain.

Local Care: Begin by gently removing any skin debris or secretions from the ear canal using a dry cotton bud or small piece of dry cotton wool. Ear irrigation with 0.9% sodium chloride may be performed only if the tympanic membrane is fully visible and intact (no perforation). Otherwise, irrigation should be avoided.

Antibiotic Therapy: For bacterial infection, ciprofloxacin ear drops are recommended for 7 days:

Children ≥ 1 year: 3 drops in the affected ear, twice daily.

Adults: 4 drops in the affected ear, twice daily.
If a foreign body is identified, it should be removed carefully during the examination.

Acute Otitis Media (AOM)
Acute otitis media (AOM) is an infection that causes inflammation in the middle ear, typically triggered by viral or bacterial pathogens. It is most common in children under the age of 3, though it occurs less frequently in adults. The primary bacterial agents involved in AOM include Streptococcus pneumoniae, Haemophilus influenzae, Moraxella , and, in older children, Streptococcus pyogenes.

Clinical Features
Symptoms: AOM typically presents with a rapid onset of ear pain. In infants, this may manifest as crying, irritability, difficulty sleeping, and reluctance to nurse. Fever and ear discharge (otorrhoea) are common, and additional symptoms like rhinorrhoea, cough, diarrhea, or vomiting may also be present. These symptoms may complicate the diagnosis,

highlighting the importance of examining the tympanic membrane.

Otoscopy Findings: Key findings on otoscopy include a bright red or, if a rapture is imminent, a yellowish tympanic membrane. Pus may be visible, either externalized (draining into the ear canal if the membrane has ruptured) or internalized (indicating an opaque or bulging tympanic membrane). The presence of these signs, combined with ear pain or fever, supports the diagnosis of AOM.

Differential Diagnosis

A red tympanic membrane alone, without bulging or perforation, suggests viral otitis, particularly in the context of an upper respiratory infection, or may result from prolonged crying or high fever.

Air bubbles or fluid behind an intact tympanic membrane, without signs of acute infection, suggests otitis media with effusion (OME), not AOM.

Complications

Complications are more common in high-risk children, including those with malnutrition, immunodeficiency, or ear malformations. These complications may include chronic suppurative otitis media, mastoiditis, brain abscess, or meningitis.

Treatment

Pain and Fever Management: Paracetamol is recommended for the management of pain and fever, as outlined in Chapter 1.

Ear Irrigation: Contraindicated in cases of tympanic membrane rupture or when the membrane cannot be fully visualized. Ear drops are generally not recommended.

Antibiotic Therapy

Antibiotics are warranted in the following cases:

Children under 2 years old.

Children showing signs of severe infection (e.g., vomiting, fever >39°C, severe pain).

Children are at higher risk for complications (e.g., malnutrition, immunodeficiency, ear malformation).

For other children:

Watchful Waiting: If the child can be re-evaluated within 48 to 72 hours, delaying antibiotic therapy is preferred. Most cases resolve spontaneously with symptomatic management (pain and fever control).

Antibiotic Prescription: If symptoms do not improve or worsen within 48 to 72 hours, antibiotics should be prescribed. If the child cannot be re-examined, antibiotics should be started immediately.

Reevaluation: If the child is on antibiotics, caregivers should be instructed to return if symptoms persist after 48 hours.

First-Line Antibiotic Treatment

Amoxicillin is the first-line treatment:

Children: 30 mg/kg, three times daily (maximum 3 g daily) for 5 days.

Adults: 1 g, three times daily for 5 days.

Alternatively, Amoxicillin/Clavulanic Acid (Co-amoxiclav) can be used:

Children <40 kg: 25 mg/kg, twice daily for 5 days.

Children ≥40 kg and adults:

Ratio 8:1: 2000 mg daily (2 tablets of 500/62.5 mg, twice daily).

Ratio 7:1: 1750 mg daily (1 tablet of 875/125 mg, twice daily).

Management of Ear Drainage

If ear drainage persists without fever or pain, and the child has otherwise improved (e.g., reduced systemic symptoms and local inflammation), there is no need to change the antibiotic regimen. The ear canal can be cleaned with gentle dry mopping until no further drainage is observed.

Alternative Antibiotic Option

Azithromycin: For children over 6 months, 10 mg/kg once daily for 3 days.

Chronic Suppurative Otitis Media (CSOM)

Chronic Suppurative Otitis Media (CSOM) is a persistent bacterial infection of the middle ear characterized by continuous purulent (pus-filled) discharge through a perforated tympanic membrane. This condition is often the result of long-term or inadequately treated ear infections.

Causative Organisms

The main bacterial pathogens associated with CSOM include

Pseudomonas aeruginosa, Proteus species, Staphylococcus species, and various Gram-negative and anaerobic bacteria.

Clinical Features

Symptoms: The hallmark feature of CSOM is a persistent purulent discharge lasting for more than two weeks. This discharge is typically accompanied by hearing loss, which may progress to partial or complete deafness. Notably, CSOM often occurs without significant pain or fever, which distinguishes it from acute infections.

Otoscopy Findings: Otoscopic examination typically reveals a perforated tympanic membrane along with the presence of purulent exudate.

Complications

Superinfection (Acute Otitis Media, AOM): If a patient with CSOM suddenly develops fever and ear pain, this could indicate a superinfection (AOM). In such cases, antibiotics should be prescribed to manage the acute infection.

Mastoiditis: New onset of high fever, severe ear pain, or tenderness behind the ear in a patient with CSOM could suggest mastoiditis, a severe complication that may require hospitalization and prompt treatment.

Brain Abscess or Meningitis: In rare cases, the infection can spread beyond the ear, causing severe complications such as brain abscess or meningitis. Symptoms may include impaired consciousness, neck stiffness, and focal neurological signs, such as facial nerve paralysis. These conditions require urgent medical attention.

Treatment

Ear Canal Care: Gently remove any secretions from the ear canal using a dry cotton bud or a small piece of dry cotton wool. Avoid traumatic cleaning, as it may worsen the condition.

Antibiotic Therapy: Ciprofloxacin ear drops are typically recommended for treating CSOM. They should be applied until no further drainage is observed (usually around two weeks, but can extend to a maximum of four weeks if necessary):

Children (≥1 year): 3 drops, twice daily
Adults: 4 drops, twice daily
Complications Management
Chronic Mastoiditis: This is a medical emergency. It requires immediate hospitalization and prolonged antibiotic therapy to cover the common pathogens associated with CSOM. The treatment regimen typically includes:
Ceftriaxone IM for 10 days
Ciprofloxacin PO for 14 days
Atraumatic cleaning of the ear canal should be performed under medical supervision, and surgical intervention may be necessary in some cases.
If transfer to a hospital is required, the first dose of antibiotics should be administered before transfer.
Meningitis: In cases where there are signs of meningitis, such as altered consciousness, neck stiffness, or neurological deficits, immediate treatment in a hospital setting is essential.
Conclusion
CSOM is a chronic condition that can lead to serious complications if not adequately managed. Early

identification of symptoms and prompt treatment with appropriate antibiotics can help reduce the risk of more severe infections like mastoiditis and meningitis. Regular follow-up care is crucial to monitor for any changes in the patient's condition.

Whooping Cough (Pertussis)

Whooping cough, or pertussis, is a highly contagious bacterial infection of the lower respiratory tract caused by Bordetella pertussis. The infection spreads primarily through respiratory droplets released when infected individuals cough or sneeze.

While pertussis can affect individuals of all ages, it is most severe in infants and young children, particularly those who are not vaccinated or incompletely vaccinated. Adolescents and adults may experience milder symptoms, often leading to delayed recognition of the infection, which increases the risk of transmission, especially to vulnerable infants.

Clinical Features

Pertussis progresses in three stages:
1. Incubation Period: The incubation period lasts 7-10 days before symptoms appear.
2. Catarrhal Phase (1 to 2 weeks): This phase is characterized by mild symptoms resembling a common upper respiratory infection, including a runny nose (coryza) and a cough. During this stage, it can be difficult to distinguish pertussis from other respiratory infections.
3. Paroxysmal Phase (1 to 6 weeks): This is the most distinctive phase, where the patient experiences prolonged coughing spells lasting at least two weeks. These coughing fits are often followed by a characteristic "whoop" sound during inhalation. In some cases, the coughing fits may lead to vomiting. Fever is either absent or mild, and between coughing episodes, the physical exam typically appears normal. However, patients may experience increasing fatigue.
Atypical Presentations:
Infants under 6 months: In this age group, coughing bouts may

be less pronounced, and the patient may experience apnea (pauses in breathing) and cyanosis (bluish skin due to lack of oxygen). The characteristic "whoop" sound may not be present.

Adults: In adults, the cough may persist for a prolonged period, but other symptoms are often absent or less severe.

4. Convalescent Phase: Symptoms gradually resolve, typically over several weeks to months, though coughing may persist for some time.

Complications

Major Complications:

Secondary bacterial pneumonia: This can occur in infants, and the presence of new-onset fever may indicate its development.

Malnutrition and dehydration: Caused by poor feeding due to coughing and vomiting.

Neurological complications: These can include seizures, encephalopathy (brain dysfunction), and, in rare cases, sudden death.

Minor Complications:

Subconjunctival hemorrhage (bleeding in the eyes), petechiae (small, pinpoint red spots), hernias, and rectal prolapse can occur due to the intense coughing.

Management and Treatment

Hospitalization: Infants under 3 months of age and children with severe cases should be hospitalized. Infants under 3 months must be closely monitored for apnea and other complications, ideally with 24-hour supervision.

Outpatient Care: Parents of children treated as outpatients should be educated on warning signs that require re-consultation, such as:

Fever
Worsening general condition
Dehydration or malnutrition
Apnea or cyanosis

Isolation:

Respiratory isolation is crucial until the patient has completed 5 days of antibiotic treatment. This helps prevent the spread of the infection to others, especially those who are unvaccinated.

Home Isolation: Avoid contact with infants who have not been vaccinated or have incomplete vaccinations.

Hospital Isolation: Suspected pertussis cases should be isolated in a single room or grouped with other pertussis cases, away from other patients.
Hydration and Nutrition:
Ensure that children under 5 years of age remain well-hydrated. Breastfeeding should continue, with small, frequent feedings recommended after coughing bouts and vomiting.
Weight monitoring is essential throughout the illness, and food supplements may be required during the recovery phase to support growth and nutrition.
Antibiotic Treatment
First-line Antibiotics:
Azithromycin (oral, for 5 days) is the recommended antibiotic for pertussis treatment.
Children: 10 mg/kg once daily (max. 500 mg/day).
Adults: Day 1: 500 mg, Days 2-5: 250 mg once daily.
Alternative Antibiotics:
Co-trimoxazole (oral, for 14 days) can be used if macrolides are contraindicated or not tolerated. However, it is not recommended for infants under 1

month of age or during the last month of pregnancy.

Erythromycin is another option, though azithromycin is better tolerated due to its shorter treatment duration and fewer doses per day.

Post-exposure Prophylaxis

All individuals in close contact with a confirmed or suspected pertussis case should receive post-exposure prophylaxis. Pertussis vaccination should be updated for both the patient and contacts. If the primary vaccination series is incomplete, it should be finished, not restarted.

Prevention

Vaccination: Routine vaccination is essential for the prevention of pertussis. Vaccines containing pertussis antigens, such as DTP (diphtheria, tetanus, and pertussis) or DTP combined with hepatitis B (DTP-Hep B) or Haemophilus influenzae type B (DTP-Hib-Hep B), are administered starting at 6 weeks of age, following the national immunization protocol.

Booster Doses: Since neither vaccination nor natural infection provides lifelong immunity, booster doses are necessary to reinforce immunity and reduce the risk of transmission, especially to young children.

Conclusion

Pertussis remains a serious and preventable disease, especially in infants and young children. Early diagnosis, appropriate antibiotic treatment, and effective isolation practices are crucial to controlling its spread. Vaccination is the cornerstone of prevention, but boosters are essential to maintaining immunity throughout life.

Bronchitis

Bronchitis is the inflammation of the bronchial tubes, classified into two types:

Acute Bronchitis

Acute bronchitis is a short-term inflammation, often caused by viral infections or irritants. Symptoms include a persistent cough, mucus production, wheezing, and mild chest discomfort. It usually resolves within a few weeks with supportive care such as rest, hydration, and cough remedies.

Chronic Bronchitis

Chronic bronchitis is a long-term condition, commonly caused by smoking or environmental pollutants. It is characterized by a productive cough lasting for at least three months per year for two consecutive years. Treatment focuses on symptom management, including medications and smoking cessation, to prevent further lung damage.

Acute Bronchitis

Acute bronchitis is the inflammation of the bronchial mucosa, typically caused by viral infections, though Mycoplasma pneumoniae may be a contributing factor in older children. In children over 2 years, recurrent cases or wheezing bronchitis might indicate asthma. For infants under 2 years, bronchiolitis should be considered.

Clinical Features:

The illness often starts with rhinopharyngitis, which progresses to pharyngitis, laryngitis, and tracheitis. Key symptoms include:

Dry cough at the beginning, followed by productive cough

Low-grade fever (without tachypnea or dyspnea)
Bronchial wheezing on pulmonary auscultation
Treatment:
Children: Amoxicillin, 30 mg/kg, 3 times daily (max 3 g/day) for 5 days
Adults: Amoxicillin, 1 g, 3 times daily for 5 days
Supportive care includes maintaining hydration, humidifying the air, and using paracetamol for fever management.
Nasal irrigation with 0.9% sodium chloride or Ringer lactate is recommended for children to clear airways.
Antibiotics are typically unnecessary in patients with viral infections unless they present with severe symptoms or underlying conditions (e.g., malnutrition, severe anemia, or cardiac disease). Antibiotics may be necessary if there's evidence of a secondary bacterial infection, such as Haemophilus influenzae or Streptococcus pneumoniae.
Chronic Bronchitis

Chronic bronchitis involves long-term inflammation of the bronchial mucosa, primarily due to factors like tobacco smoke, air pollution, allergies (asthma), or repeated acute bronchitis episodes. It may lead to chronic obstructive pulmonary disease (COPD).

Clinical Features:

Chronic bronchitis is diagnosed by a productive cough lasting at least three months per year for two consecutive years. In the early stages, patients may not experience dyspnea, but as the condition progresses, exertional shortness of breath becomes evident. The following signs may be present:

Wheezing upon pulmonary auscultation (tuberculosis must be ruled out)

Increased sputum production, often purulent

Onset or worsening of dyspnea over time

Treatment:

Antibiotics are generally not effective for chronic bronchitis itself but may be indicated during acute exacerbations, particularly in patients with poor general health.

Smoking cessation and avoiding irritants are essential components of management.

Long-term management focuses on improving lung function and preventing further deterioration, potentially involving bronchodilators or corticosteroids.

Bronchiolitis

Bronchiolitis is an acute viral infection of the lower respiratory tract, predominantly affecting children under 2 years of age. It is primarily caused by respiratory syncytial virus (RSV), responsible for up to 70% of cases. Transmission occurs via respiratory droplets or contact with contaminated surfaces.

Clinical Features:

Initial symptoms: Rhinopharyngitis and dry cough, which may develop into more severe symptoms like wheezing and difficulty breathing.

Severity indicators: Increased respiratory rate, signs of respiratory distress (e.g., nasal flaring, sternal retractions), or cyanosis. In severe cases, oxygen levels may drop below 92%.

Treatment:

Outpatient management: Focuses on symptomatic care, such as maintaining hydration, using nasal saline irrigation, and managing fever.

Hospitalization is required in severe cases with criteria like significant respiratory distress, cyanosis, or respiratory rate above 60/min. Children may also need supplemental oxygen or, in rare cases, nasogastric feeding if they are too fatigued to feed orally.

Bronchodilators are sometimes used on a trial basis for severe respiratory distress. If effective, they may be continued; otherwise, treatment is discontinued.

Antibiotics are not recommended unless there is a risk of secondary bacterial infection (e.g., pneumonia).

Prevention:

Proper hand hygiene is critical, as RSV is most commonly transmitted through hands. Health care workers should wear appropriate protective gear, including gowns, gloves, and surgical masks, when interacting with affected children. Cohorting patients to reduce cross-contamination is also recommended.

In conclusion, the management of bronchiolitis and bronchitis involves a combination of supportive care and targeted interventions based on severity and underlying conditions. Careful monitoring and early intervention are crucial, particularly in high-risk populations.

Acute Pneumonia is an infection of the pulmonary alveoli caused by viruses, bacteria (e.g., Streptococcus pneumoniae, Haemophilus influenzae, Staphylococcus aureus, or atypical bacteria), or parasites (e.g., Pneumocystis).

In children under 5 years, pneumonia may present with rapid onset and severe symptoms.

In children over 5 years and adults, the condition can vary, with symptoms often including fever, cough, and difficulty breathing.

Persistent pneumonia refers to cases where symptoms do not improve with initial treatment, requiring further evaluation and management.

Pneumonia in Children Under 5 Years of Age

Etiology: The most common causes of pneumonia in children under 5 years are viral infections, Streptococcus pneumoniae, and Haemophilus influenzae.

Clinical Features:

Respiratory Rate (RR) Guidelines:

Children under 1 month: RR $\geq$ 60 breaths/minute

Children 1 to 11 months: RR $\geq$ 50 breaths/minute

Children 12 months to 5 years: RR $\geq$ 40 breaths/minute

General Symptoms:

Cough, difficulty breathing, and fever (often high, but can be low-grade or absent, which may indicate a severe condition).

Tachypnea (increased RR) often occurs.

Pulmonary auscultation may show dullness, decreased breath sounds, crepitations, or bronchial breathing.

Severe Signs of Pneumonia include:
Chest indrawing (visible retraction of the chest wall on inspiration)
Cyanosis (blueness around lips, mucosa, or nails, or SpO2 < 90%)
Nasal flaring, altered consciousness, stridor, grunting, and refusal to feed.
For children under 2 months, moderate chest indrawing is normal due to flexible thoracic walls.
Treatment:
Severe Pneumonia (Inpatient Care):
In children under 2 months, treatment typically includes a combination of IV ampicillin and gentamicin for 5 to 10 days. If the condition does not improve after 48 hours, cloxacillin may be added.
For children 2 months to 5 years, first-line treatment includes IV ceftriaxone or ampicillin with gentamicin for 3 days. If necessary, cloxacillin is added for 48 hours if there is no improvement.
For Children 0-7 Days:

If the child is less than 2 kg, ampicillin and gentamicin are given every 12 hours. For children ≥ 2 kg, these are administered every 8 hours.

Follow-up and Adjustments:

After 3 days of improvement, the treatment may switch to oral amoxicillin, and antibiotics should continue for a total of 10 to 14 days.

If there's no improvement, additional antibiotics like azithromycin are considered, especially for atypical pneumonia or if tuberculosis is suspected.

Adjuvant Therapy:

If oral feeding is not possible, nasogastric tubes are used. Intravenous fluids are given to maintain hydration, especially in children with severe respiratory distress. Oral rehydration solutions (ORS) are used as needed.

Management in Non-severe Cases:

Children with no signs of severe pneumonia can be treated as outpatients, except for infants. Amoxicillin (30 mg/kg three times daily) is given for 5 days.

Follow-up is crucial within 48-72 hours to monitor progress, especially if the child's condition worsens.

Additional Considerations:

For malnourished children, respiratory rate thresholds may be lowered by 5 breaths/minute.

Conditions like malaria, staphylococcal pneumonia, and tuberculosis should be considered based on the child's symptoms and exposure history.

Pneumonia in Children (Over 5 Years) and Adults

Pneumonia is a common respiratory infection that can be caused by a variety of pathogens. The primary etiological agents in both children over 5 years of age and adults are viruses, Streptococcus pneumoniae (pneumococcus), and Mycoplasma pneumoniae. The management approach differs based on the severity of the condition and the age of the patient.

Clinical Features

Pneumonia often presents suddenly with high fever (above 39°C), thoracic pain, and oral herpes lesions in cases of pneumococcal infection. These signs, along with nonspecific symptoms such as abdominal pain and meningeal symptoms, may make the diagnosis difficult, especially in children.

Severe pneumonia is characterized by the following signs:

Respiratory distress: Tachypnea (rate > 30 breaths/min), intercostal or subclavicular indrawing, and nasal flaring.

Cyanosis: Bluish discoloration of lips, oral mucosa, or fingernails.

Altered consciousness: Drowsiness or confusion.

Tachycardia: Heart rate > 125 beats/minute.

Dullness or abnormal auscultation findings: Decreased vesicular breath sounds, localized crepitations, or bronchial wheeze.

High-risk patients include:

Elderly individuals.

Patients with heart failure, sickle cell disease, or severe chronic bronchitis.

Those who are immunocompromised (e.g., severe malnutrition, HIV with CD4 count <200).

Treatment of Severe Pneumonia

For severe pneumonia requiring inpatient care, initial antibiotic therapy should be administered parenterally, followed by oral treatment as the patient's condition improves:

1. Ceftriaxone (IM or slow IV):
Children: 50 mg/kg once daily.
Adults: 1 g once daily.

Treatment should continue intravenously for at least 3 days, then transition to oral amoxicillin once clinical improvement is noted:
Children: 30 mg/kg 3 times daily (max. 3 g daily).
Adults: 1 g 3 times daily.

Alternatively, ampicillin (IV or IM) can be used:
Children: 50 mg/kg every 6 hours.
Adults: 1 g every 6-8 hours.

If the patient's condition worsens or does not improve within 48 hours, Ceftriaxone should be combined with cloxacillin (IV infusion):
Children: 25-50 mg/kg every 6 hours.
Adults: 2 g every 6 hours.

After 3 days of clinical improvement with no fever,

treatment should switch to amoxicillin/clavulanic acid (co-amoxiclav) for 10-14 days:
Children (< 40 kg): 50 mg/kg twice daily.
Children (≥ 40 kg) and adults: 3000 mg daily in two doses.
If tuberculosis (TB) is suspected but not yet confirmed, continue treatment with ceftriaxone + cloxacillin while awaiting results. In case TB is ruled out, azithromycin may be added for suspected atypical pneumonia.

Treatment for Non-Severe Pneumonia (Outpatient Care)
For less severe cases, oral antibiotics are typically used:
Amoxicillin:
Children: 30 mg/kg 3 times daily (max. 3 g daily) for 5 days.
Adults: 1 g 3 times daily for 5 days.
Follow-up is necessary in 48-72 hours to assess the response to treatment. If symptoms worsen or fail to improve, consider adding azithromycin for atypical pneumonia.

Persistent Pneumonia
In cases where pneumonia does not improve with standard treatment, consider other

diagnoses such as atypical pneumonia or tuberculosis.
For atypical pneumonia, antibiotics targeting Mycoplasma pneumoniae or Chlamydophila pneumoniae are recommended:
Azithromycin (PO):
Children: 10 mg/kg (max. 500 mg) once daily for 5 days.
Adults: 500 mg on day 1, then 250 mg daily for the next 4 days.
Alternatives include:
Erythromycin or doxycycline (except in pregnant or breastfeeding women).

Staphylococcal Pneumonia

Staphylococcus aureus is a common cause of severe pneumonia in young children, especially those in poor health (e.g., malnutrition). It is also a complication in measles.
Clinical signs include:
High fever or hypothermia.
Shock symptoms.
Skin lesions (entry points for the bacteria).
Respiratory distress: Tachypnea, dry cough, or abnormal lung auscultation.
Chest x-rays may show multilobar consolidation, pneumatoceles, or spontaneous

pneumothorax. Immediate antibiotic therapy is critical:
1. Ceftriaxone (IM or slow IV): 50 mg/kg once daily.
2. Cloxacillin (IV): Administered over 60 minutes, as per pediatric dosing guidelines.
After 3 days of clinical improvement, switch to amoxicillin/clavulanic acid or clindamycin (IV or PO) for 10-14 days, depending on the severity.

Summary of Key Treatment Steps:
1. Initial treatment for severe pneumonia with ceftriaxone and, if necessary, cloxacillin.
2. Outpatient treatment for less severe cases with amoxicillin.
3. Follow-up after 48-72 hours to reassess and adjust treatment based on clinical response.
4. Persistent pneumonia may require a reassessment for atypical infections or tuberculosis.

By maintaining a thorough and vigilant approach, healthcare providers can ensure that pneumonia is effectively managed in children and adults, reducing the risks of complications and long-term morbidity.

Asthma

Asthma is a chronic inflammatory disease of the airways, characterized by airway hyperresponsiveness, leading to recurrent episodes of wheezing, shortness of breath, chest tightness, and coughing. These episodes are typically linked to airflow obstruction in the lungs, which is often reversible either spontaneously or with treatment.

Triggers for asthma exacerbations include allergens, infections, physical activity, medications (e.g., aspirin), and tobacco use. Symptoms can be more pronounced at night.

In children under 5 years, asthma-like symptoms are usually associated with respiratory infections, with symptom-free intervals between episodes. Over time, wheezing tends to become less frequent, and most children in this age group do not go on to develop chronic asthma.

Asthma can be classified into two types:

1. Acute Asthma (Asthma Attack): Sudden worsening of asthma symptoms due to triggers or inflammation.
2. Chronic Asthma: Ongoing, persistent inflammation and airway narrowing leading to recurrent symptoms.

Acute Asthma (Asthma Attack)

Last updated: June 2023

An asthma attack refers to the sudden worsening of asthma symptoms, which can vary in both intensity and duration. These exacerbations are often unpredictable.

Assessment of Severity

Rapid assessment of the asthma attack's severity is essential and is determined by the following clinical criteria. Not all signs may be present simultaneously.

For Children Over 2 Years and Adults:

Mild to Moderate Attack:

Patient can speak in full sentences.

Slight increase in respiratory rate (RR) and heart rate (HR).

$SpO_2 \geq 90\%$ ($\geq 92\%$ for children 2-5 years).

No signs of severe or life-threatening attack.

Severe or Life-Threatening Attack:
Patient unable to speak in full sentences.
Very high RR (children 2-5 years: > 40/min; children > 5 years and adults: > 30/min).
Very high HR (children 2-3 years: > 180/min; children 4-5 years: > 150/min; children > 5 years and adults: > 120/min).
SpO2 < 90% (or < 92% for children 2-5 years).
Signs of life-threatening attack such as altered consciousness, exhaustion, silent chest, cyanosis, arrhythmia, or hypotension.

Treatment

Mild to Moderate Attack:
1. Reassure the patient and monitor their response to treatment.
2. Treatment approach:
Salbutamol (100 µg/puff): 2–10 puffs every 20 minutes for the first hour using a metered-dose inhaler (MDI).
Ipratropium MDI (20 µg/puff): 4-8 puffs every 20 minutes for the first hour.

Prednisolone (oral): 1-2 mg/kg (maximum 50 mg) for children over 5 years and adults.
Administer oxygen if SpO2 < 94%.
If the attack resolves:
Observe for at least 1 hour (4 hours if the patient lives far from the healthcare center).
For follow-up treatment, administer Salbutamol MDI every 4–6 hours for 24–48 hours and Prednisolone daily for up to 5 days.
If only partially resolved:
Continue Salbutamol MDI every 1–4 hours.
If symptoms recur in children up to 5 years, administer Prednisolone again.
If the attack does not improve or worsens, escalate to severe attack treatment.
Severe or Life-Threatening Attack:
1. Position the patient in a semi-sitting posture.
2. Treatment approach:
Oxygen to maintain SpO2 between 94% and 98%.
Nebulizer solutions:
For children < 5 years: Salbutamol (2.5 mg) +

Ipratropium (0.25 mg) every 20 minutes for the first hour.
For children 5–11 years: Salbutamol (2.5–5 mg) + Ipratropium (0.5 mg) every 20 minutes for the first hour.
For children ≥ 12 years and adults: Salbutamol (5 mg) + Ipratropium (0.5 mg) every 20 minutes for the first hour.
Prednisolone (oral): 1-2 mg/kg (maximum 50 mg).
If oral medication is unavailable, consider Dexamethasone (0.15–0.6 mg/kg for children) or Hydrocortisone IV (4 mg/kg for adults).
If no improvement after 1 hour, transfer to intensive care, continue oxygen, and start Magnesium sulfate (2 g for adults or 40 mg/kg for children) by IV infusion over 20 minutes.
Pregnancy Considerations:
Treatment in pregnant women is the same as for adults, with the addition of oxygen to reduce the risk of fetal hypoxia in mild or moderate attacks.
Additional Considerations:
Always assess for underlying lung infections and treat

appropriately, regardless of the attack's severity.

Chronic Asthma

Clinical Features

Chronic asthma is characterized by recurrent respiratory symptoms such as wheezing, shortness of breath, and chest tightness, which vary in frequency and intensity. These symptoms can disrupt daily activities and cause disturbed sleep. In some cases, asthma symptoms may be triggered by exercise or specific allergens.

Treatment Approach

Long-term management of asthma includes the use of inhaled corticosteroids (ICS) and long-acting beta-2 agonists (LABA). LABAs should always be combined with ICS and never used alone. Combination inhalers are preferred when available.

Short-acting beta-2 agonists (SABA) like Salbutamol can be used for symptom relief.

Severity-Based Treatment for Children Over 6 Years and Adults

Treatment is initiated based on the severity of asthma, which is

re-evaluated and adjusted as needed.
Intermittent Asthma:
Daytime symptoms < 2 times per month.
Salbutamol when symptomatic.
Beclometasone/Formoterol when symptomatic (alternative to salbutamol).
Mild Persistent Asthma:
Daytime symptoms ≥ 2 times monthly, affecting daily activities.
Beclometasone (low dose) daily, with Salbutamol for symptoms.
Moderate Persistent Asthma:
Daytime symptoms most days or nighttime symptoms ≥ once weekly.
Beclometasone (low dose) + Salmeterol daily, with Salbutamol for symptoms.
Severe Persistent Asthma:
Daily daytime symptoms or frequent nighttime symptoms.
Beclometasone (medium dose) + Salmeterol daily, with Salbutamol for symptoms.
Dosage and Medication Adjustment
The goal is to find the lowest effective dose to manage symptoms while minimizing

adverse effects. Beclometasone (MDI) should not exceed 2000 micrograms per day.

Additional Considerations

For children, a spacer should be used with inhalers, and patients should be educated on inhaler techniques and recognizing asthma attack symptoms. Management may need to be adjusted based on the patient's age, symptoms, and response to treatment.

References

1. Global Initiative for Asthma (2022). Global Strategy for Asthma Management and Prevention: 2022 Update. Available at: https://ginasthma.org/gina-reports/ [Accessed on 23 January 2023].

2. World Health Organization (2022). Pocket Book of Primary Health Care for Children and Adolescents: Guidelines for Health Promotion, Disease Prevention, and Management from the Newborn Period to Adolescence. WHO Regional Office for Europe.

Pulmonary Tuberculosis

Pulmonary tuberculosis (TB) is a bacterial infection caused by Mycobacterium tuberculosis, which primarily spreads through the inhalation of respiratory droplets from an infected individual. After initial exposure, the bacteria multiply slowly within the lungs. In most cases, the infection resolves on its own or remains dormant. However, only around 10% of infected individuals develop active tuberculosis. The likelihood of progressing to active disease is elevated in individuals with weakened immune systems. In some regions, approximately 50% of new TB cases are co-infected with HIV.

For additional details on tuberculosis, refer to the Tuberculosis guide by Médecins Sans Frontières (MSF).

Clinical Features

In regions where TB is common, the condition should be considered in any patient presenting with respiratory symptoms lasting longer than two weeks, particularly if they do not respond to non-specific antibacterial treatments.

Laboratory Diagnosis

The Xpert® MTB/RIF test, which simultaneously detects M. tuberculosis and rifampicin resistance in sputum, is recommended for diagnosis. In settings where this test is unavailable, sputum smear microscopy can be performed. For patients with suspected HIV co-infection, additional diagnostic tests like the lateral flow urine lipoarabinomannan assay (LF-LAM) should be considered.

Treatment

The standard treatment for pulmonary tuberculosis consists of a six-month regimen with a combination of four antituberculosis medications: isoniazid, rifampicin, pyrazinamide, and ethambutol. The treatment is divided into two phases: the initial phase and the continuation phase. If drug-resistant TB is detected, treatment duration is extended and alternative drug combinations are used.

Successful treatment requires strict adherence to the prescribed regimen to ensure complete recovery and prevent the development of drug resistance. Both the patient and the healthcare provider must be committed to the treatment process, and it is crucial that patients receive proper case management until their treatment is finished.

Prevention

BCG Vaccination: Administered to neonates, BCG vaccination offers around 59% protection against pulmonary tuberculosis.

Infection Control: In healthcare settings, standard precautions and airborne precautions should be implemented for suspected or confirmed TB cases.

Preventive Therapy for Close Contacts: Individuals in close contact with active TB patients should receive isoniazid preventive therapy for six months.

Differential Diagnosis

The symptoms of pulmonary tuberculosis, such as prolonged cough, fever, weight loss, and fatigue, can be similar to those of other conditions, including pneumonia, chronic obstructive pulmonary disease (COPD), lung cancer, pulmonary distomatosis (parasitic infections), and melioidosis (in Southeast Asia).

References

1. World Health Organization (2018). Global Tuberculosis Report 2018. Available at: https://apps.who.int/iris/handle/1 0665/274453 [Accessed 21 October 2019].
2. Global Laboratory Initiative (2018). GLI Model TB Diagnostic Algorithms. Available at: http://www.stoptb.org/wg/gli/ass ets/documents/GLI_algorithms.p df [Accessed 21 October 2019].
3. World Health Organization (2018). Weekly Epidemiological Record/Relevé Épidémiologique Hebdomadaire. 93(8), 73–96. Available at: https://www.who.int/immunizati on/policy/position_papers/bcg/en / [Accessed 21 October 2019].

Chapter 3

Gastrointestinal disorders

This chapter addresses several important gastrointestinal disorders commonly encountered in clinical practice, highlighting their identification and initial management:

Acute Diarrhea: Discusses its causes, symptoms, and the need for prompt rehydration and investigation to identify the underlying condition.
Shigellosis: Examines the bacterial infection caused by Shigella, its transmission, clinical presentation, and the importance of antibiotic treatment.
Amoebiasis: Focuses on the parasitic infection caused by Entamoeba , its symptoms, diagnostic methods, and effective anti-amoebic treatment.
Disorders of the Stomach and Duodenum: Reviews common conditions such as gastro-oesophageal reflux disease (GERD), gastric and duodenal ulcers, and dyspepsia, emphasizing diagnostic approaches and management strategies.
Gastro-oesophageal Reflux: Explores the causes and symptoms of GERD, along with treatment options including lifestyle changes and medications.
Gastric and Duodenal Ulcers in Adults: Investigates the pathophysiology of ulcers,

focusing on risk factors like H. pylori infection and NSAID use, and the necessary treatment protocols.
Dyspepsia: Reviews the causes of upper abdominal discomfort, its differential diagnosis, and the management of symptoms associated with functional and organic disorders.
Stomatitis: Addresses the inflammation of the mouth lining, its causes, and the management of pain and infection based on the underlying etiology.
Oral and Oropharyngeal Candidiasis: Discusses the diagnosis and treatment of oral thrush caused by Candida, emphasizing antifungal therapy.
Oral Herpes: Explores the herpes simplex virus infection, its presentation as oral sores, and the use of antiviral medications to manage outbreaks.
Other Infectious Causes: Highlights various other infections that can affect the oral and gastrointestinal systems, with a focus on their diagnosis and specific treatments.

Stomatitis from Scurvy (Vitamin C Deficiency): Reviews the clinical presentation of scurvy, its oral manifestations, and the role of vitamin C supplementation in treatment.

Other Lesions Resulting from Nutritional Deficiency: Examines how deficiencies in vitamins and minerals contribute to oral lesions, and the importance of nutritional correction for recovery.

Acute Diarrhea: Overview and Management

Definition and Clinical Features: Acute diarrhea is characterized by the passage of at least three liquid stools per day lasting less than two weeks. The condition is commonly divided into two clinical types:

1. Diarrhea without blood: Often caused by viral infections (e.g., rotavirus, enterovirus), bacterial infections (e.g., Vibrio cholerae, enterotoxigenic Escherichia coli, Salmonella, Yersinia enterocolitica), or parasitic infections (e.g., giardiasis). This type may also be associated with conditions like malaria,

respiratory infections, and otitis media.

2. Diarrhea with blood: Typically caused by bacterial infections (e.g., Shigella, Campylobacter , enterohemorrhagic E. coli, Salmonella) or parasitic infections (e.g., Entamoeba).

Diagnosis and Clinical Signs:

Key symptoms to assess include:

Profuse watery diarrhea: Common in cases of cholera and enterotoxigenic E. coli infections.

Repeated vomiting: Often seen in cholera.

Fever: Suggestive of infections like salmonellosis or viral diarrhea.

Blood in stool: Associated with bacterial infections like shigellosis or amoebiasis.

In children, severe and rapid dehydration warrants suspicion of cholera, especially in the presence of watery diarrhea.

Treatment Principles:

1. Rehydration: The most critical aspect of managing acute diarrhea, especially to prevent dehydration and malnutrition. Oral rehydration solution (ORS) should be administered,

particularly between feedings in children. In cases of severe dehydration, intravenous fluids may be necessary.

2. Zinc Supplementation: Zinc has been shown to reduce the duration and severity of diarrhea and prevent future episodes in the following dosages:

Children under 6 months: 10 mg once daily for 10 days.

Children 6 months to 5 years: 20 mg once daily for 10 days.

Zinc is administered in combination with ORS, dissolving tablets in water and given as a single spoonful to the child.

3. Malnutrition Prevention: Continue a normal diet for affected children, with increased breastfeeding frequency for infants. While breastfeeding is encouraged, ORS should still be administered separately from breastfeeds.

4. Avoid Anti-Diarrheal Medications: These should not be used routinely as they may delay the resolution of the condition. Anti-emetics and anti-diarrhoeal drugs should also be

avoided unless specifically indicated.

Antimicrobial Treatment:
Diarrhea without blood: Most viral causes do not require antibiotics. However, antibiotics are recommended for specific cases like cholera or giardiasis.
Diarrhea with blood: For suspected shigellosis, first-line antibiotic therapy is warranted, as amoebiasis is less common and typically requires antiparasitic treatment only if Entamoeba is confirmed.

Prevention Strategies:
Breastfeeding: Exclusive breastfeeding is critical in reducing both the severity of diarrhoeal episodes and the risk of mortality.
Hygiene and Sanitation: Ensuring clean water access and promoting handwashing with soap, especially before eating and after defecation, significantly reduces diarrhea transmission.
Vaccination: In regions with high mortality rates from rotavirus, WHO recommends routine rotavirus vaccination for children aged 6 weeks to 24 months.

Conclusion:

Effective management of acute diarrhea relies on preventing dehydration through rapid fluid and electrolyte replacement, zinc supplementation to reduce symptom severity, and appropriate treatment for underlying infections. Prevention strategies focused on improved hygiene, breastfeeding, and vaccination are key to reducing incidence and mortality associated with diarrhoeal diseases.

References
1. World Health Organization (WHO). Weekly Epidemiological Record. 1st February 2013, 88th Year, No. 5, 2013, 88, 49–64. Available at: https://www.who.int/wer/2013/wer8805.pdf [Accessed 02 January 2019].

Shigellosis
Shigellosis is a highly contagious bacterial infection characterized by bloody diarrhea. It is caused by four different species of Shigella: S. , S. , S. , and S. . Among these, S. type 1 (Sd1) is the most concerning, as it is responsible for large-scale outbreaks and carries the highest

case fatality rate, up to 10%. Certain groups, including children under 5, malnourished individuals, post-measles children, and adults over 50, are at higher risk for severe outcomes.

Clinical Features

Shigellosis presents with abdominal pain, frequent and painful bowel movements, and bloody diarrhea, often accompanied by fever. Severe cases may result in complications like febrile seizures (5-30% in children), rectal prolapse (3%), septicemia, intestinal obstruction, and, in severe cases, hemolytic uremic syndrome. A rapid onset of fever (above 39°C), signs of dehydration, altered mental status, and seizures should prompt immediate clinical attention, particularly in patients with risk factors for severe disease.

Diagnosis and Laboratory Testing

Diagnosis is confirmed through stool culture, with antibiotic sensitivity testing to guide treatment. Shigella strains can develop antibiotic resistance quickly, so ongoing monitoring through monthly cultures and sensitivity testing is critical, especially during outbreaks.

Treatment Protocols

1. First-line Treatment

Ciprofloxacin (oral) for 3 days: 15 mg/kg twice daily for children (max 1 g/day), 500 mg twice daily for adults.

If the strain is resistant or no improvement is seen within 48 hours, alternative treatments such as ceftriaxone (intramuscular) or azithromycin (oral) are recommended:

Ceftriaxone: 50-100 mg/kg for children (max 1 g/day), 1-2 g daily for adults, for severe infections or when oral administration is not feasible.

Azithromycin: 12 mg/kg on day 1 and 6 mg/kg once daily from days 2-5 for children; 500 mg on day 1, then 250 mg daily for adults.

If no improvement occurs after 48 hours, consider treating for amoebiasis.

2. Supportive Care

Rehydration: Oral rehydration solution (ORS) should be administered as per WHO guidelines, especially to prevent dehydration (see Dehydration, Chapter 1).

Nutritional support: Provide nutritional supplements and maintain a high-calorie intake (2500 kcal/day during hospitalization, 1000 kcal/day for outpatients).

Zinc supplementation for children under 5 years to help reduce the severity and duration of diarrhea.

Avoid using antidiarrheal medications like loperamide, as they can worsen the condition by slowing peristalsis.

Complications Management

If complications like rectal prolapse or septic shock occur, they must be managed appropriately (see respective chapters). Severely ill patients should be admitted to the hospital, and isolation procedures should be enforced. Preventive measures such as handwashing, food hygiene, and proper food storage are essential to control the spread of the infection.

Epidemic Context

In epidemic situations, additional caution is necessary, including isolation of patients, exclusion of infected children from school, and enhanced hygiene practices. Epidemic management also involves early identification and rapid treatment to limit the spread.

References

1. Kotloff, K.L., et al. Seminar: Shigellosis. The Lancet, Volume 391, Issue 10122, 801-812, February 24, 2018.
2. World Health Organization. Pocket book for hospital care in children: guidelines for the management of common childhood illnesses, 2013. Available at: WHO [Accessed 20 September 2018].

Amoebiasis

Amoebiasis is an intestinal parasitic infection caused by Entamoeba . It is primarily transmitted through the fecal-oral route by ingesting cysts present in contaminated food or water. Although most individuals (approximately 90%) infected with E. remain asymptomatic, a minority (10%) develop symptomatic disease.

Types of Amoebiasis

1. Intestinal Amoebiasis (Amoebic Dysentery)
Pathogenic amoebae can penetrate the colonic mucosa, leading to amoebic dysentery, which presents similarly to shigellosis—a primary cause of dysentery.

2. Extra-intestinal Amoebiasis
In some cases, the amoebae migrate via the bloodstream to form peripheral abscesses. The most common extraintestinal manifestation is an amoebic liver abscess.

Clinical Features
Intestinal Amoebiasis (Amoebic Dysentery)
Diarrhea with visible red blood and mucus.
Abdominal pain and tenesmus.
Absence or low-grade fever.
Dehydration may occur, depending on severity.

Amoebic Liver Abscess
Painful hepatomegaly (enlarged liver), sometimes with mild jaundice.
Symptoms of anorexia, weight loss, nausea, and vomiting.
Fever (often intermittent), sweating, chills, and general malaise.

Diagnostic Investigations
1. Amoebic Dysentery
Confirmed by identifying E. trophozoites in fresh stool samples.
Presence of cysts alone does not confirm active disease.
2. Amoebic Liver Abscess
Diagnosed using serological tests like indirect hemagglutination or ELISA.
Imaging: Conduct an EFAST (Extended Focused Assessment with Sonography for Trauma) examination, specifically evaluating the liver and spleen for abscess-like lesions. Seek expert consultation, if necessary, for interpretation.

Treatment Protocols
Amoebic Dysentery
Antiparasitic Medications:
Tinidazole (oral):
Children: 50 mg/kg once daily for 3 days (maximum 2 g/day).
Adults: 2 g once daily for 3 days.
Metronidazole (oral):
Children: 15 mg/kg three times daily for 5 days.
Adults: 500 mg three times daily for 5 days.
Supportive Care:

Use oral rehydration salts (ORS) to prevent or manage dehydration as per WHO protocols (see Dehydration, Chapter 1).
Note: If laboratory facilities are unavailable, initial treatment should target shigellosis. Treat for amoebiasis only if symptoms persist after adequate treatment for shigellosis.

Amoebic Liver Abscess
Antiparasitic Medications:
Tinidazole (oral): Same dosage as for amoebic dysentery, continued for 5 days.
Metronidazole (oral): Same dosage as for amoebic dysentery but extended for 5–10 days.

Footnote
(a) POCUS should only be conducted and interpreted by trained professionals to avoid misdiagnosis of amoebic abscesses as other liver pathologies.

Key Considerations
Effective treatment hinges on distinguishing E. from non-pathogenic strains.
In settings without laboratory confirmation, empiric treatment strategies should align with

clinical presentation and response to initial therapy.
Public health measures like improved sanitation, safe drinking water, and hygiene education are critical in preventing amoebiasis outbreaks.

References

1. World Health Organization. Pocket book for hospital care in children: guidelines for the management of common childhood illnesses, 2013. Accessible at: WHO [Accessed: 20 September 2018].
2. Stanley, S.L. Amoebiasis. The Lancet, Volume 361, Issue 9362, 1025–1034, March 22, 2003.

Stomach and Duodenal Disorders

This section addresses common conditions affecting the stomach and duodenum, focusing on their diagnosis and management:

Gastroesophageal Reflux Disease (GERD): Covers the causes, symptoms, and treatment options for reflux-related issues.

Gastric and Duodenal Ulcers in Adults: Discusses the etiology, clinical presentation, and therapeutic approaches for peptic ulcer disease.

Dyspepsia: Highlights the evaluation and management of indigestion and related gastrointestinal discomfort.

Disorders of the Stomach and Duodenum

Gastroesophageal Reflux Disease (GERD)

Clinical Features:
GERD typically presents with burning epigastric pain or heartburn, which is often alleviated by antacids. Acid regurgitation, particularly in postural positions like leaning forward or lying down, is a hallmark symptom. In the absence of dysphagia or signs of esophageal stenosis, these symptoms are generally benign.

Treatment:
1. Lifestyle Modifications:
Advise patients to eliminate alcohol and tobacco use.
2. Medications:
First-line therapy: Aluminum hydroxide/magnesium hydroxide combination (400 mg/400 mg), 1-2 tablets orally three times daily, taken 20-60 minutes post-meal or during pain episodes.
Second-line therapy: If antacids are insufficient, prescribe

omeprazole (20 mg orally once daily in the morning) for 3 days.

3. In Children: Avoid pharmacological treatment; instead, encourage rest and elevate the sleeping position to 30-45 degrees.

Caution:

Aluminum hydroxide/magnesium hydroxide can interfere with the absorption of medications like ciprofloxacin, doxycycline, and iron salts. Spacing medication intake appropriately is essential to minimize interactions.

Gastric and Duodenal Ulcers

Clinical Features:

Patients often report burning epigastric pain or cramps that occur between meals or awaken them at night. Symptoms are episodic, lasting several days, and may be accompanied by nausea or vomiting. Major complications include perforation and gastrointestinal bleeding.

Management of Non-Complicated Ulcers:

Avoid NSAIDs and aspirin in patients with ulcers or a history of ulcers.

Initiate treatment with omeprazole (20 mg orally once daily in the morning for 7-10 days). For severe or recurrent cases, increase the dose to 40 mg once daily for up to 8 weeks.

Consider Helicobacter pylori (H. pylori) eradication therapy if recurrent ulcer symptoms necessitate prolonged anti-ulcer treatment.

Management of Complications:

1. Perforation:

Suspect perforation in patients with acute, severe epigastric pain and abdominal rigidity.

Begin immediate fluid resuscitation with Ringer's lactate and pain management.

Administer intravenous omeprazole (40 mg daily) and broad-spectrum antibiotics.

Refer for surgical intervention if possible; otherwise, continue conservative management with IV hydration and antibiotics.

2. Gastrointestinal Bleeding:

Black stools (melena) or hematemesis suggest bleeding. Most cases resolve spontaneously.

For stable patients: Maintain hydration and keep NPO for 12 hours.
For active bleeding or hemodynamic instability: Initiate IV fluids, insert a nasogastric tube, and consult a specialist.
H. pylori Eradication Therapy:
Administer omeprazole (20 mg twice daily), clarithromycin (500 mg twice daily), and amoxicillin (1 g twice daily) for 7 days.
For penicillin-allergic patients, replace amoxicillin with metronidazole (500 mg twice daily).
Note: Persistent symptoms after treatment warrant evaluation for gastric malignancy.

Dyspepsia

Clinical Features:
Dyspepsia is characterized by epigastric discomfort or pain after meals, often accompanied by bloating, fullness, and nausea. Functional dyspepsia is diagnosed after ruling out organic causes such as GERD, ulcers, drug-induced symptoms, or gastric cancer.
Treatment:

1. Investigate and treat underlying causes, including intestinal parasitic infections.
2. For H. pylori-positive patients, follow eradication guidelines.
3. In H. pylori-negative cases, omeprazole (10 mg orally once daily) for 4 weeks may relieve symptoms.

Clinical Guidelines

Clinical guidelines recommend managing dyspepsia with a case-based approach, incorporating evidence-based therapy and diagnostic evaluation for underlying conditions.

Stomatitis

Overview:

Stomatitis refers to inflammation of the oral mucosa, caused by infections (fungal, viral, bacterial), nutritional deficiencies, or trauma. In severe cases, it can lead to dehydration or malnutrition, especially in children.

Management:
1. Maintain hydration and offer non-irritating, soft foods.
2. Ensure oral hygiene to prevent recurrence.
3. Treat underlying infections or deficiencies:

Oral candidiasis: Use nystatin oral suspension (1 ml four times daily for 7 days) or miconazole oral gel.

Oral herpes: For severe cases or immunocompromised patients, administer acyclovir (200 mg five times daily for children under 2 years; 400 mg five times daily for older children and adults).

Both conditions require monitoring for complications and addressing any secondary infections.

Key Considerations:

Evaluate for systemic illnesses like HIV in recurrent or severe cases.

Avoid triggering factors like acidic foods and poor oral hygiene.

Other Infectious Causes

For additional infectious etiologies, refer to the discussions in:

Pharyngitis: See Chapter 2 for an overview of common pathogens, clinical presentation, and treatment strategies.

Diphtheria: Refer to Chapter 2 for diagnostic criteria,

complications, and management guidelines.

Measles: Explore Chapter 2 for insights into epidemiology, clinical features, and supportive care recommendations.

Stomatitis Due to Scurvy (Vitamin C Deficiency)

Clinical Features

Scurvy-associated stomatitis is characterized by bleeding gums and may be accompanied by lower limb pain in infants, typically caused by subperiosteal hemorrhage. This condition is often observed in populations experiencing poor nutritional quality, such as those reliant on food aid in refugee camps or other resource-limited settings.

Treatment

Ascorbic Acid (Vitamin C) Administration:
The optimal therapeutic dose of vitamin C for treating scurvy has not been definitively established. The following dosage recommendations are based on age and clinical guidelines:

For children aged 1 month to 11 years:
100 mg orally, three times daily.

For children 12 years and older, as well as adults:
250 mg orally, three times daily.
Alternatively:
For children aged 1 month to 3 years:
100 mg orally, twice daily.
For children aged 4 to 11 years:
250 mg orally, twice daily.
For children 12 years and older, as well as adults:
500 mg orally, twice daily.
Duration of Treatment:
Vitamin C therapy should be continued for at least two weeks or until symptoms resolve. Following this initial phase, a preventive daily dose is recommended to address ongoing nutritional deficits:
Children and adults: 50 mg daily, administered for as long as the nutritional deficiency persists.
Notes:
Timely administration of vitamin C effectively resolves symptoms and prevents recurrence. Early recognition of scurvy's hallmark clinical features is essential in high-risk populations to ensure prompt treatment and improve outcomes.

Oral Lesions Caused by Nutritional Deficiencies

Overview

Various vitamin and mineral deficiencies can lead to oral lesions, manifesting as angular stomatitis or glossitis, which can impair eating and exacerbate nutritional deficiencies if untreated.

Causes and Features

1. Vitamin Deficiencies:

Vitamin B2 (Riboflavin):
Deficiency may cause angular stomatitis (cracks and sores at the corners of the mouth) and glossitis (inflammation of the tongue).

Niacin (Vitamin B3):
Associated with oral manifestations seen in Pellagra, which include glossitis and stomatitis (refer to Pellagra, Chapter 4).

Vitamin B6 (Pyridoxine):
Deficiency can result in glossitis, stomatitis, and cheilitis (inflammation of the lips).

2. Iron Deficiency:
Commonly causes angular stomatitis and is often linked to conditions such as anemia (refer to Anaemia, Chapter 1).

Treatment Strategy

Vitamin and Mineral Replacement Therapy:
Administer therapeutic doses of the specific deficient vitamin or mineral, tailored to the individual's needs based on clinical assessment.

Multivitamins: Although beneficial for general health, they are inadequate for addressing severe or clinical vitamin deficiencies, as therapeutic doses far exceed the amounts provided in standard multivitamin formulations.

Evidence-Based Approach

Recognition and Diagnosis:
Evaluate clinical signs of oral lesions and consider dietary history to identify potential deficiencies.

Laboratory tests can confirm specific deficiencies when available.

Management:
Prompt initiation of curative doses improves symptoms and prevents complications.

Concurrent dietary education helps reduce recurrence, particularly in at-risk populations.

Early intervention and targeted treatment of nutritional deficiencies are critical in reversing lesions and restoring overall health.

Chapter 4
Dermatological Conditions

This chapter delves into a wide range of skin disorders, categorizing them by etiology and clinical presentation. The focus includes:

1. Parasitic Infestations:
Scabies and lice, common parasitic skin conditions, their transmission, clinical manifestations, and management.

2. Fungal Infections:
Exploration of superficial fungal diseases affecting the skin, nails, and hair, with emphasis on diagnosis and antifungal therapies.

3. Bacterial Infections:
Detailed insights into impetigo, furuncles, carbuncles, erysipelas, cellulitis, and cutaneous anthrax, including their pathogenic causes and treatment approaches.

4. Endemic Treponematoses:
Discussion of regional treponemal infections like yaws and pinta, highlighting

epidemiology and therapeutic interventions.

5. Leprosy:
Coverage of Mycobacterium infection, focusing on its skin and systemic manifestations, diagnosis, and strategies for disease control.

6. Viral Dermatology:
Examination of herpes simplex and herpes zoster (shingles), with guidance on antiviral treatments and symptom management.

7. Other Skin Disorders:
Analysis of conditions such as eczema, seborrheic dermatitis, urticaria, and pellagra, emphasizing their pathophysiology, diagnostic criteria, and evidence-based treatments.

Dermatology: A Case-Based Overview

Skin diseases, particularly those of infectious origin, are highly prevalent and often indicate broader public health issues. A significant incidence of such conditions in a population may point to inadequate water supply and poor hygiene.

Clinical Approach to Skin Diseases

1. Importance of Dermatological Examination

Patients frequently seek care late in the disease process, by which time primary lesions may be obscured by secondary infections. To ensure accurate diagnosis and treatment:

Address secondary infections first.

Reevaluate the patient to identify the primary skin condition.

2. Classification of Skin Lesions

Careful observation of lesion types is crucial for diagnosis:

Macule: Flat, non-palpable discoloration differing from surrounding skin.

Papule: Small, circumscribed, slightly raised, solid lesion (< 1 cm).

Vesicle and Bulla: Fluid-filled blisters, vesicles (< 1 cm) and bullae (> 1 cm).

Pustule: Vesicle containing pus.

Nodule: Firm, elevated lesion (> 1 cm), extending into the dermis or subcutaneous tissue.

Erosion: Epidermal loss that heals without scarring.

Excoriation: Erosion caused by scratching.

Ulcer: Loss of epidermis and dermis that results in scarring.
Scale: Detaching flakes of epidermis.
Crust: Dried serum, blood, or pus on the skin's surface.
Atrophy: Thinning of the skin.
Lichenification: Thickened skin with enhanced natural markings.

3. Distribution and Arrangement of Lesions

Observe the lesion's body distribution and arrangement:
Patterns may be isolated, clustered, linear, or annular (ring-shaped).
Note if the lesions cause itching.

4. Identifying Potential Triggers

Investigate possible causes, such as:
Insect bites.
Parasitic skin infections (e.g., scabies, lice).
Contact with irritants like plants, animals, metals, or detergents.

5. Treatment History and Risk Factors

Assess any ongoing or previous treatments (topical, oral, or injectable).
Evaluate local or systemic signs such as secondary infections,

fever, lymphangitis, or septicemia.

6. Environmental and Family Conditions

Analyze family hygiene and sanitary conditions, especially for contagious diseases like scabies, lice, or scalp ringworm.

7. Vaccination Status

Confirm tetanus immunization to prevent complications from secondary infections or trauma to lesions.

Evidence-Based Practice

A structured and meticulous dermatological assessment facilitates accurate diagnosis and targeted therapy, addressing both individual treatment needs and the underlying public health determinants contributing to skin disease prevalence.

Scabies: A Comprehensive Review

Scabies, caused by the Sarcoptes scabiei hominis mite, is a parasitic skin condition that presents in two forms: ordinary scabies and crusted scabies (Norwegian scabies). Ordinary scabies is generally mild and moderately contagious, while crusted scabies is highly contagious, difficult to treat, and often associated with immunodeficiency.

Transmission and Public Health Considerations

Transmission occurs primarily through direct skin contact and, less frequently, via shared clothing or bedding. Effective management necessitates simultaneous treatment of the affected individual and their close contacts, along with decontamination of clothing and bedding to interrupt the transmission cycle.

Clinical Features

Ordinary Scabies

Older Children and Adults:

Symptoms: Intense nocturnal itching, often indicative of scabies when shared by close contacts.

Lesions:

Scabies burrows: Wavy lines (5–15 mm) representing mite tunnels, commonly found in interdigital spaces, wrist flexors, areolae, buttocks, elbows, and axillae. The back and face are typically spared.

Entry vesicles: Small vesicles marking the mite's entry points.

Scabies nodules: Persistent reddish-brown nodules, especially on male genitalia, not necessarily indicating active infection post-treatment.

Secondary lesions: Resulting from scratching (excoriations) or bacterial superinfection (e.g., impetigo).

Infants and Young Children:
Often presents with vesicular eruptions, particularly on the palms, soles, back, and face.

Secondary infections and eczema are common.

Scabies nodules may appear in axillae as isolated symptoms.

Examining the caregiver's hands may assist in diagnosis.

Crusted (Norwegian) Scabies
This severe form manifests as thick, scaly, erythematous plaques, often mimicking psoriasis. It may or may not cause itching (50% of cases). Delay in diagnosis can result in outbreaks.

Treatment
General Management
1. Simultaneous Treatment: Treat all close contacts, regardless of symptom presence.

2. Decontamination: Wash clothing and bedding at ≥60°C, dry in direct sunlight, or seal in plastic bags for 72 hours.

Ordinary Scabies

1. Topical Scabicides:

Apply over the entire body, including the scalp, postauricular areas, palms, soles, and umbilicus. Avoid mucous membranes, inflamed skin, or breastfeeding women's breasts. Reapply if the product is washed off.

Preferred Treatment:

Permethrin 5% cream: Single application with an 8-hour contact period, repeated after seven days.

Benzyl benzoate 25% lotion: Requires dilution based on age and application guidelines.

2. Oral Therapy:

Ivermectin (200 mcg/kg): Effective as a single dose or repeated after seven days to minimize treatment failure risk. Contraindicated in children <15 kg and pregnant women.

3. Special Considerations:

Treat secondary bacterial infections 24–48 hours before scabicide application.

Persistent itching post-treatment may not indicate treatment failure but could suggest residual inflammation or an alternate condition.

Crusted Scabies

1. Combination Therapy:

Oral ivermectin and topical scabicides administered weekly for 2–3 weeks or more, depending on severity.

Remove crusts with salicylic acid ointment before applying topical treatments for better efficacy.

2. Infection Control:

Isolate the patient to prevent environmental spread through exfoliated skin scales.

Use personal protective equipment (PPE) for healthcare staff.

Decontaminate the environment (bedding, floors, and surfaces).

Monitoring Treatment Effectiveness

Persistent itching for 1–3 weeks post-treatment is typical and not indicative of failure.

Reevaluate if symptoms persist beyond four weeks, as this may suggest reinfestation or improper treatment (e.g., missed scalp

application or hand washing during treatment).
Persistent burrows warrant retreatment of the patient and contacts.

Special Precautions
In endemic areas for Loa loa, ivermectin administration must be preceded by microfilaraemia assessment due to potential severe neurological complications. Topical treatments are preferred in such cases.

Summary
Successful scabies management relies on a comprehensive approach encompassing accurate diagnosis, effective treatment, simultaneous management of contacts, and meticulous environmental decontamination. Prompt identification and intervention are critical in preventing outbreaks, especially for crusted scabies.

Lice (Pediculosis): Overview and Management
Pediculosis is a parasitic infestation caused by three species of lice specific to humans: head lice, body lice, and pubic lice. While generally

benign, the condition is highly contagious and spreads through direct or indirect contact. Body lice can serve as vectors for serious diseases such as relapsing fever, typhus, and trench fever.

Clinical Features

Head Lice:

Predominantly affects children. Common symptoms include itching and scratch marks, particularly at the nape of the neck and around the ears. Prolonged infestations may lead to secondary infections, such as impetigo. Diagnosis involves detecting live lice or viable nits (shiny, gray) attached to hair shafts within 5 mm of the scalp.

Body Lice:

Typically associated with populations living in poor conditions, such as refugees, prisoners, or the homeless. Symptoms include itching, scratch marks (notably on the back, beltline, and armpits), and inflamed or infected skin lesions. Lice and nits are often found on clothing rather than directly on the body.

Pubic Lice:

Considered a sexually transmitted infection (STI), pubic lice infestations cause itching and scratch marks in the pubic and perianal areas. Other hairy regions, such as the armpits, thighs, and eyelashes, may also be affected. Diagnosis involves finding lice and nits at the base of hair shafts, although they may be less visible.

General Management Principles
Examination of Contacts:
Identify and examine close contacts to prevent re-infestation. For body lice, assess for systemic infections, and for pubic lice, screen for other STIs.
Hygiene and Environmental Measures:
Decontaminate personal items, such as combs, clothing, and bedding, to prevent the spread. Effective methods include:
Wash items in hot water (≥60°C) for at least 30 minutes.
Ironing or sun-drying.
Sealing unwashed items in plastic bags for two weeks.
Treatment Strategies
Head Lice
Topical Treatments:
4% Dimeticone Lotion:

Suitable for children over 6 months and adults.
Apply to dry hair, ensuring coverage of the nape and areas behind the ears. Leave for 8 hours, then rinse thoroughly.
Avoid flames or heat sources during application due to ignition risks.
1% Permethrin Lotion:
Recommended for children over 2 months and adults.
Leave on hair for 10 minutes before rinsing.
Repeat treatment after 7 days to eliminate any newly hatched lice.
Decontamination:
Treat all personal items in contact with the scalp. Avoid unnecessary treatment of individuals with non-viable (dull, white, >1 cm from the scalp) nits.
Body Lice
Mass Treatment:
Apply 0.5% permethrin powder directly to the inside of clothing and undergarments in contact with the skin.
Rub the powder in thoroughly and leave for 12–24 hours.
Treat all clothing, headwear, and bedding by sealing them in a

plastic bag with permethrin powder. Repeat after 8–10 days if needed.

Pubic Lice

Topical Treatment:
Shave or apply 1% permethrin lotion to affected areas, following head lice application guidelines.
Treat sexual partners simultaneously to prevent reinfestation.

Environmental Measures:
Decontaminate clothing and bedding as described for head lice.

Additional Considerations

Secondary Bacterial Infections:
If present, initiate systemic antibiotic therapy (e.g., for impetigo) 24–48 hours before starting local antiparasitic treatments. Ensure patients tolerate the antiparasitic agent before applying it to the affected area.

Superficial Fungal Infections

Superficial fungal infections are common and generally mild conditions affecting the skin, scalp, and nails. They are caused by either Candida albicans or dermatophytes and can manifest in various forms based on the site of infection.

Clinical Features and Treatment Approaches

Candidiasis

1. Candidal Diaper Dermatitis

Symptoms: Redness and peeling of the perianal area, sometimes accompanied by pustules. Secondary bacterial infections may occur in severe cases.

Management:

Keep the area clean and dry using regular soap and water.

Reduce moisture by allowing air exposure or changing diapers frequently.

Apply zinc oxide ointment if diarrhea is present.

Persistent or severe cases may indicate intestinal involvement; oral nystatin (100,000 IU, four times daily for 20 days) may be prescribed.

2. Candidiasis of Skin Folds

Symptoms: Moist, red, and irritated areas in skin folds.

Treatment: Apply miconazole 2% cream twice daily for 2–4 weeks.

3. Oral and Vulvovaginal Candidiasis

Refer to specific guidelines (e.g., for stomatitis or abnormal vaginal discharge).

Dermatophytosis (Ringworm)

Dermatophyte infections vary depending on the affected site, such as the scalp, smooth skin, skin folds, or nails.

Scalp Infections

Tinea Capitis (Scalp Ringworm):
Symptoms: Scaly, red patches with broken hair ends; severe cases (kerion) may cause pus-filled lesions and swollen lymph nodes. Chronic cases (favus) can lead to permanent hair loss.

Treatment:
Local care: Clean affected areas with soap and water, dry, and apply miconazole 2% cream or Whitfield's ointment twice daily for at least 2 weeks.
Systemic antifungal therapy (required for full resolution):
Griseofulvin:
Children (1–12 years): 10–20 mg/kg/day (max 500 mg).
Adults: 500–1000 mg/day.
Duration: 6–12 weeks.
Itraconazole:
Children: 3–5 mg/kg/day (max 200 mg).

Adults: 200 mg/day for 2–4 weeks.
Treat secondary bacterial infections (e.g., impetigo) before initiating antifungal therapy.
Pain management: Paracetamol.
Pregnancy: Avoid oral antifungals; use topical treatments to control infection until oral options become feasible postpartum.

Skin Infections (Tinea Corporis and Tinea Cruris)

1. Tinea Corporis (Body Ringworm):
Symptoms: Itchy, red, scaly patches with a distinct raised border and central clearing.
Treatment:
Local therapy for mild cases: Miconazole 2% cream or Whitfield's ointment twice daily for 2–4 weeks.
Extensive infections: Griseofulvin (4–6 weeks) or itraconazole (2 weeks).

2. Tinea Cruris (Groin Infection):
Symptoms: Itchy, red patches in the groin area, often with pustules along the edges.
Treatment: Apply miconazole 2% cream twice daily. Avoid

Whitfield's ointment for lesions in sensitive areas.

Fungal Infections of Skin Folds and Feet

1. Tinea Pedis (Athlete's Foot):
Symptoms: Itchy, peeling skin, typically in the spaces between the third and fourth toes.
Treatment: Regular application of miconazole 2% cream.

2. Candidal Intertrigo:
Symptoms: Red, macerated patches in interdigital spaces, especially the first and second toes.
Treatment: Similar to tinea pedis, with miconazole as the primary agent.

Nail Infections (Onychomycosis)
Symptoms: Thickened, discolored, and brittle nails.
Treatment: Oral antifungal therapy, such as griseofulvin, for 12–18 months. However, long treatment durations often lead to challenges in adherence and frequent relapses.

General Recommendations
1. Decontaminate combs, bedding, and clothing by washing at ≥60°C, ironing, or sealing items in plastic bags for 2 weeks.

2. Simultaneously treat close contacts to prevent reinfection.
3. Address secondary infections (if present) before starting antifungal therapy.

Case-Based Evidence

Case 1: A 3-year-old with scalp ringworm and kerion responded well to systemic griseofulvin combined with miconazole cream.

Case 2: A 45-year-old with tinea pedis managed with topical miconazole showed complete resolution within 3 weeks.

Scope of Bacterial Skin Infections

Bacterial skin infections cover a range of conditions caused by various bacteria, primarily Staphylococcus aureus and Streptococcus pyogenes. These infections can present from mild, localized issues to severe, widespread conditions. Early detection, proper management, and antibiotic treatment are crucial to preventing complications and promoting healing.

Impetigo

Impetigo is a highly contagious superficial skin infection,

typically caused by Staphylococcus aureus or Streptococcus pyogenes. It manifests as red sores that burst and form a yellowish-brown crust. It primarily affects children, requiring topical or, in severe cases, oral antibiotics for treatment. Good hygiene practices help control its spread.

Furuncles and Carbuncles

Furuncles (boils) and carbuncles are infections of the hair follicles, most commonly caused by Staphylococcus aureus. Furuncles appear as painful, pus-filled lumps, while carbuncles are larger clusters of boils that may cause fever. Both require drainage and, in some cases, systemic antibiotics, especially if caused by antibiotic-resistant bacteria like MRSA.

Erysipelas and Cellulitis

Erysipelas and cellulitis are bacterial infections affecting the skin's deeper layers. Erysipelas is a superficial infection caused by Streptococcus pyogenes, marked by well-defined red, swollen areas. Cellulitis, often caused by both Streptococcus pyogenes and Staphylococcus aureus, involves deeper tissues and presents with diffuse redness and swelling. Both require prompt antibiotic therapy to prevent systemic spread and complications.

Impetigo: A Detailed Overview
Impetigo is a superficial and contagious skin infection primarily caused by Streptococcus pyogenes (group A ß-haemolytic streptococcus) and Staphylococcus aureus. Co-infection with both bacteria is common, and the infection spreads through direct contact. Factors like poor hygiene and a lack of access to water can exacerbate the spread of the infection. Impetigo typically affects children but can also complicate preexisting dermatoses in adults, such as lice, scabies, eczema, herpes, and chickenpox.

Clinical Features of Impetigo
Non-bullous Impetigo (Classic Form): This form begins as a flaccid vesicle on erythematous (red) skin, which later becomes pustular and forms a yellowish crust. Multiple stages of infection may occur simultaneously within

the same lesion, but typically, these lesions do not leave permanent scarring. The most common sites for infection include the nose, mouth, limbs, and scalp.

Bullous Impetigo: This type is characterized by large, flaccid bullae (blisters) and skin erosions, often affecting the anogenital region in newborns and infants.

Ecthyma: A more severe form of impetigo that presents as ulcerative lesions, typically leaving scars. Ecthyma is more commonly seen in immunocompromised individuals (e.g., those with HIV), as well as in diabetics and alcoholics.

Systemic Features: Typically, impetigo does not cause fever or systemic symptoms. However, severe complications, including abscess formation, cellulitis, lymphangitis, osteomyelitis, septicemia, and acute glomerulonephritis, may occur. It is important to monitor for signs of glomerulonephritis after infection.

Treatment of Impetigo

1. Localized Non-Bullous Impetigo (fewer than five lesions in one area):

First-line Treatment: Clean affected areas with soap and water, then apply 2% mupirocin ointment three times a day for seven days. After three days, reassess the infection. If there is no improvement, switch to oral antibiotics.

Prevention: Keep fingernails short, avoid touching the lesions, and cover them with gauze to minimize spread.

2. Extensive Non-Bullous Impetigo (more than five lesions or multiple areas affected), Bullous Impetigo, Ecthyma, or in Immunocompromised Patients:

Initial Management: Clean the infected areas two to three times daily with soap and water and keep nails short. Abscesses, if present, should be incised.

Oral Antibiotics:

Cefalexin (7-day course):

Neonates under 7 days: 25 mg/kg twice daily

Neonates 7-28 days: 25 mg/kg three times daily

Children (1 month–12 years): 25 mg/kg twice daily

Children over 12 years and adults: 1 g twice daily
Cloxacillin (7-day course):
Children over 10 years: 15 mg/kg three times daily (max 3 g daily)
Adults: 1 g three times daily
Note: For newborns with lesions around the umbilicus, administer cloxacillin intravenously.

3. Penicillin-Allergic Patients:
If the patient is allergic to penicillin and resistant to macrolides, azithromycin is recommended for three days. The dosing regimen is:
Children: 10 mg/kg once daily
Adults: 500 mg once daily

Additional Considerations
School Quarantine: Children with impetigo should be kept away from school until they have received 24–48 hours of appropriate antibiotic therapy.
Underlying Conditions: Evaluate and treat any underlying dermatosis such as lice, scabies, eczema, herpes, or fungal infections like scalp ringworm, as these conditions may exacerbate impetigo.
Contact Tracing: It is crucial to identify and treat contacts who

may have been exposed to the infection.

Post-Infection Monitoring: Three weeks after the infection, check for proteinuria (using a urine dipstick test) to screen for potential complications like glomerulonephritis.

Furuncles and Carbuncles: A Comprehensive Overview

Furuncles and carbuncles are localized infections of the hair follicle and surrounding tissue, typically caused by Staphylococcus aureus. These conditions can occur when there is necrotizing inflammation in the perifollicular area. Key risk factors for developing these infections include nasal carriage of S. aureus, skin trauma (such as breaks or maceration), poor hygiene, and systemic factors like diabetes, malnutrition, iron deficiency, and immunodeficiency.

Clinical Features

1. Furuncle: A furuncle (or boil) is a painful, red, and warm nodule that usually forms around a hair follicle. It often develops a central pustule and, as it progresses, becomes fluctuant

(filled with pus). Once it discharges purulent exudate, a core of pus is expelled, and the lesion typically heals with a depressed scar. Furuncles are commonly found on the thighs, groin, buttocks, armpits, neck, and back. These lesions do not usually present with fever.

2. Carbuncle: A carbuncle is a more severe, clustered form of furuncles, where multiple boils are interconnected. Carbuncles can cause systemic symptoms such as fever and peripheral lymphadenopathy (swollen lymph nodes). Like furuncles, they can leave a depressed scar upon healing.

Treatment

1. For a Single Furuncle:

Initial Care: Clean the affected area with soap and water twice daily, and cover with a dry dressing.

Warm Compresses: Apply warm, moist compresses to the lesion to encourage drainage and promote healing.

Post-Drainage Care: Once the furnace drains, clean the area and continue applying a dry dressing until the wound heals.

2. For Facial Furuncles, Multiple Furuncles, Carbuncles, or Immunocompromised Patients:
Local Care: Continue with the same approach as for a single furnace (cleaning, applying compresses, and dressing).
Systemic Antibiotics: Administer a 7-day course of oral antibiotics:
Cefalexin:
Neonates (under 7 days): 25 mg/kg twice daily
Neonates (7 to 28 days): 25 mg/kg three times daily
Children (1 month–12 years): 25 mg/kg twice daily
Children over 12 years and adults: 1 g twice daily
Amoxicillin/Clavulanic Acid (Co-amoxiclav):
Children < 40 kg: 25 mg/kg twice daily
Children ≥ 40 kg and adults:
8:1 ratio formulation: 2000 mg daily (two 500/62.5 mg tablets, twice daily)
7:1 ratio formulation: 1750 mg daily (one 875/125 mg tablet, twice daily)
3. For Penicillin-Allergic Patients:
Clindamycin can be used as an alternative antibiotic:

Children: 10 mg/kg three times daily
Adults: 600 mg three times daily

General Recommendations for All Patients

Hygiene: Frequent handwashing is essential to prevent the spread of infection.

Bedding: Ensure that bedding is regularly washed, as it may harbor bacteria.

Erysipelas and Cellulitis: Overview, Diagnosis, and Treatment

Erysipelas and cellulitis are acute skin infections typically caused by bacteria, most commonly Group A beta-hemolytic Streptococcus (GABHS) and sometimes Staphylococcus aureus, including methicillin-resistant S. aureus (MRSA). These infections occur when bacteria enter the skin through a break, often after trauma or inflammation. Risk factors for developing these infections include venous insufficiency, obesity, edema, lymphoedema, a history of erysipelas or cellulitis, immunosuppression, and conditions causing cutaneous inflammation, such as dermatosis or wounds.

Types of Infections

Erysipelas: A superficial infection involving the dermis and superficial lymphatic vessels. It typically presents as a well-demarcated red, swollen, and tender plaque, often affecting the lower extremities and face.

Cellulitis: A deeper infection affecting the deep dermis and subcutaneous tissue. It is usually associated with more widespread inflammation, which may include fever and systemic signs. It also commonly affects the lower legs and, occasionally, the face.

Clinical Signs

Erysipelas:

Well-defined, red, tender, swollen plaques.

Fever, lymphadenopathy (swollen lymph nodes), and lymphangitis (inflammation of lymphatic vessels).

Look for potential entry sites, such as bites, ulcers, wounds, eczema, or fungal infections.

Cellulitis:

Diffuse redness, warmth, and swelling.

Fever and possible systemic symptoms like malaise.
If there is intense pain out of proportion to the skin appearance, rapid progression of local signs, crepitus, skin necrosis, or a critically ill patient, consider necrotizing fasciitis, which requires urgent surgical intervention (refer to Chapter 10).

Potential Complications
Sepsis: Can progress to septic shock (see Chapter 1).
Glomerulonephritis: Occurs approximately 3 weeks after infection; urine dipstick tests for proteinuria are recommended.
Osteomyelitis and septic arthritis: May develop if the infection spreads to bones or joints.

Differential Diagnoses
Contact dermatitis: Inflammatory reaction to allergens or irritants.
Stasis dermatitis: Skin inflammation due to venous insufficiency.
Venous thrombosis: Blood clot formation in veins.
Erythema : Seen in Lyme disease.

Diagnostic and Paraclinical Investigations

Ultrasound: Used to confirm cellulitis and rule out abscesses, deep vein thrombosis, or foreign bodies.
Radiography: Helps detect foreign bodies or osteomyelitis and can reveal subcutaneous gas indicative of a necrotizing infection.
Urine Dipstick Test: Conducted 3 weeks post-infection to check for proteinuria, a sign of glomerulonephritis.
Treatment Strategies
1. General Care:
Erythema Monitoring: Mark the affected area with a pen to track the infection's progression or regression.
Rest and Elevation: Elevate the affected limb (e.g., leg) to reduce swelling.
Pain Management: Avoid NSAIDs due to the risk of worsening necrotizing fasciitis.
2. Antibiotic Therapy:
Outpatient Treatment:
Cefalexin (oral) for 7–10 days:
Children 1 month to 12 years: 25 mg/kg twice daily
Children 12 years and over, and adults: 1 g twice daily

Amoxicillin/Clavulanic acid (Co-amoxiclav) for 7–10 days:
Children < 40 kg: 25 mg/kg twice daily
Children ≥ 40 kg and adults:
8:1 formulation: 2000 mg daily (two 500/62.5 mg tablets, twice daily)
7:1 formulation: 1750 mg daily (one 875/125 mg tablet, twice daily)
Inpatient Treatment (for severe cases):
Cloxacillin (IV infusion) over 60 minutes:
Children 1 month to under 12 years: 12.5–25 mg/kg every 6 hours
Children 12 years and over, and adults: 1 g every 6 hours
Amoxicillin/Clavulanic acid (IV injection or infusion):
Children < 3 months: 30 mg/kg every 12 hours
Children ≥ 3 months: 20–30 mg/kg every 8 hours (maximum 3 g daily)
Adults: 1 g every 8 hours
If no clinical improvement after 48 hours, consider MRSA and switch to Clindamycin (IV):
Children 1 month and over: 10 mg/kg every 8 hours

Adults: 600 mg every 8 hours
3. For Penicillin-Allergic Patients:
Oral Clindamycin for 7–10 days:
Children: 10 mg/kg three times daily
Adults: 600 mg three times daily
IV Clindamycin (same dosing schedule as oral).

Hospitalization Criteria
Children under 3 months.
Critically ill patients (e.g., weak or drowsy children, those with cyanosis, hypotonia).
Debilitated patients (elderly, those with chronic conditions).
Risk of treatment non-compliance.
For all others, outpatient treatment is appropriate if the infection is uncomplicated.

Additional Notes
If erythema spreads despite treatment, it may indicate treatment failure due to MRSA or necrotizing infection.

Cutaneous Anthrax
Overview
Anthrax is an infectious disease caused by the bacterium Bacillus anthracis, which primarily affects herbivores such as sheep, goats, cattle, camels, and horses.

Humans typically contract the disease through direct contact between broken skin and infected animals or their byproducts (e.g., skins, wool, or carcasses). High-risk populations include livestock farmers and individuals handling animal products. While endemic regions include parts of Eastern Europe, Central Asia, Africa, South America, and the Mediterranean Basin, pulmonary and intestinal anthrax are other possible forms transmitted via inhalation or ingestion of contaminated meat.

Clinical Features

Cutaneous anthrax begins as a small, itchy papule on exposed skin areas like the face, neck, arms, or legs. This progresses to a pruritic vesicle that eventually ulcerates, forming a painless black eschar surrounded by swelling. Additional symptoms may include lymphangitis and regional lymphadenopathy. Severe cases may involve:
Lesions on the head or neck,
Systemic symptoms such as fever, malaise, headache, tachycardia, or hypotension,

Extensive edema or bullous lesions.

Diagnosis

Laboratory evaluation includes:
Microscopic examination with Gram staining or PCR testing from vesicular fluid.
Culture and drug susceptibility tests (less commonly available).

Management and Treatment

1. Uncomplicated Cases:
Ciprofloxacin: 15 mg/kg (maximum 500 mg) twice daily for children; 500 mg twice daily for adults.
Amoxicillin: 30 mg/kg (maximum 1 g) thrice daily for children; 1 g thrice daily for adults.

2. Severe Cases:
Intravenous (IV) antibiotics are recommended, such as:
Ampicillin: 50-65 mg/kg every 6-8 hours for children; 3-4 g every 6-8 hours for adults.
Combination therapy with Clindamycin (10-13 mg/kg every 8 hours for children; 900 mg every 8 hours for adults).
After stabilization, oral therapy should continue for a total of 14 days.

Prevention

Vaccination of livestock and proper disposal (burial or burning) of animal carcasses.
Post-exposure prophylaxis: Oral antibiotics for 10 days as per uncomplicated anthrax protocols.

Endemic Treponematoses
Overview
Endemic treponematoses encompass bacterial infections caused by treponema species other than Treponema pallidum (syphilis). These diseases, including yaws, pinta, and bejel, primarily affect populations in specific geographic regions and are transmitted through direct or indirect human contact. Although serological tests for syphilis (e.g., TPHA-VDRL) yield positive results, diagnosis relies on clinical evaluation due to the absence of definitive laboratory differentiation.

Key Clinical Features by Disease
1. Yaws (Treponema pertenue):
Common in tropical regions and primarily affects children aged 4-14.
Begins as a skin lesion (chancre) that may develop into larger, contagious lesions ().

Long-term complications include periostitis, osteitis, and disfiguring rhinopharyngitis.
2. Pinta (Treponema carateum):
Found in Latin America's tropical zones, affecting both children and adults.
Initial lesions are erythematous or scaly plaques, followed by pigmentation changes.
3. Bejel (Treponema pallidum subsp. endemicum):
Occurs in arid regions, particularly among nomadic children.
Symptoms include mucosal patches, bone destruction, and keratosis.

Treatment

Yaws: Single-dose azithromycin (30 mg/kg; maximum 2 g) or benzathine benzylpenicillin (1.2 MIU for children under 10; 2.4 MIU for others).
Pinta and Bejel: Treated similarly to yaws.
Penicillin-allergic patients: Doxycycline for 14 days (50 mg twice daily for children ≥8 years; 100 mg for adults).

Prevention

All symptomatic, asymptomatic contacts, and latent cases in

endemic areas should receive treatment to prevent transmission.

Leprosy

Overview

Leprosy, caused by Mycobacterium leprae, is a chronic bacterial infection transmitted through close and prolonged contact, often among household members. The disease predominantly affects young adults, with the majority of cases reported in Bangladesh, India, Brazil, and several African and Southeast Asian countries.

Clinical Presentation

Hypopigmented or erythematous skin lesions with sensory loss.

Enlarged and tender peripheral nerves leading to paralysis or deformities (e.g., foot drop, hand claw).

Infiltrated nodules on the face or extremities.

Classification Systems

1. Ridley-Jopling: Differentiates forms based on the immune response to M. :

Tuberculoid (localized, less contagious) to lepromatous (disseminated, highly contagious).

2. WHO Simplified Classification:
Paucibacillary: ≤5 lesions.
Multibacillary: >5 lesions.
Diagnosis
Ziehl-Neelsen staining of nasal or skin smears for acid-fast bacilli.
Clinical assessment is often sufficient in endemic regions.
Treatment
Paucibacillary: Rifampicin and dapsone.
Multibacillary: Rifampicin, dapsone, and clofazimine.

Herpes Simplex and Herpes Zoster

Herpes Simplex

Herpes simplex refers to a viral infection caused by the herpes simplex virus (HSV), which includes two types: HSV-1 and HSV-2. HSV-1 is primarily associated with oral lesions, such as cold sores, while HSV-2 typically causes genital herpes. This infection is characterized by periodic outbreaks of painful vesicular lesions, which can be accompanied by systemic symptoms like fever and malaise. The virus establishes latency in sensory ganglia, with potential reactivation triggered by stress, immunosuppression, or other factors.

Herpes Zoster (Shingles):

Herpes zoster, commonly known as shingles, results from reactivation of the varicella-zoster virus (VZV), which causes chickenpox during primary infection. Following initial infection, the virus remains dormant in dorsal root or cranial nerve ganglia and can reactivate later in life, often due to age-related or immunosuppressive conditions. Shingles presents as a painful, unilateral rash with vesicular lesions in a dermatomal distribution. It may lead to complications such as postherpetic neuralgia, particularly in older adults.

Herpes Simplex and Herpes Zoster

Herpes Simplex

Herpes simplex is a recurrent viral infection affecting the skin and mucous membranes, caused by the Herpes Simplex Virus (HSV). The clinical manifestations of recurrent lesions differ significantly from those of the primary infection.

Clinical Features:
Recurrent Herpes Labialis: Characterized by a tingling sensation preceding the appearance of clusters of vesicles on an inflamed, erythematous base. These vesicles primarily appear on the lips ("fever blisters") and around the mouth and may extend to the face. Recurrences result from the reactivation of a dormant virus acquired during the primary infection. Unlike the primary infection, recurrences are typically not associated with systemic symptoms such as fever, adenopathy, or general malaise.

Other Sites of Infection: Manifestations may also occur in other areas, such as:
Buccal mucosa, leading to stomatitis.
Genital areas, causing genital ulcers.
Eyes, with potential for severe ophthalmic complications.
Secondary bacterial infections in affected regions.
Treatment:

General Care: Clean the lesions gently with soap and water twice daily until healed.

Secondary Infections: For bacterial superinfection, treat with antibiotics as recommended for impetigo.

Herpes Zoster (Shingles)

Herpes zoster is an acute viral condition caused by the reactivation of the varicella-zoster virus (VZV). While chickenpox represents the primary infection, shingles occurs when the dormant virus reactivates, often years later.

Clinical Features:

Neurological and Dermatological Signs: Initial symptoms include unilateral neuralgic pain, which precedes the appearance of vesicles on an erythematous base. These vesicles follow the dermatomal distribution of the affected nerve pathway.

Common Sites: Lesions typically appear on the thorax but may also involve the face, increasing the risk of ophthalmic complications.

Demographics: The condition is more prevalent in adults than in children.

Treatment:
Symptomatic Management: Pain relief is central, with oral paracetamol commonly prescribed.
Antiviral Therapy: Oral acyclovir is indicated in severe cases, such as necrotic or extensive lesions or those on the face that may risk eye involvement. Early initiation within 48 hours of lesion onset is crucial.

Other Skin Disorders

Eczema

A chronic skin condition marked by redness, itching, and scaling, often triggered by irritants or allergens. Managed with emollients, topical corticosteroids, and trigger avoidance.

Seborrheic Dermatitis

A relapsing inflammatory skin disorder affecting sebaceous-rich areas like the scalp and face, characterized by greasy scales and redness. Treated with antifungal shampoos and mild corticosteroids.

Urticaria

A transient allergic reaction presenting as raised, itchy hives. Triggered by allergens or physical factors. Managed with antihistamines and trigger avoidance; severe cases require emergency care.

Pellagra

A niacin deficiency disease causing dermatitis, diarrhea, and dementia. Manifests as photosensitive, scaly patches. Treated with niacin supplementation and nutritional support.

Eczema

A chronic inflammatory condition of the skin characterized by redness, itching, and varying degrees of dryness or scaling. It may present in acute, subacute, or chronic forms, often triggered by environmental factors, allergens, or irritants.

Key Features:

Red, scaly patches with intense itching.

Lesions may weep, crust, or become lichenified over time due to chronic scratching.

Commonly affects the face, hands, and flexural areas like the elbows and knees.

Management:

Identification and avoidance of triggering factors.

Topical corticosteroids or emollients to reduce inflammation and maintain skin hydration.

Seborrheic Dermatitis

A chronic, relapsing condition affecting areas with a high density of sebaceous glands. Thought to be associated with yeast-like fungi, such as Malassezia.

Key Features:

Greasy, yellowish scales on erythematous patches, typically on the scalp (dandruff), face, and upper chest.

May cause pruritus but is often asymptomatic.

Management:

Regular cleansing with antifungal shampoos or soaps (e.g., containing ketoconazole or selenium sulfide).

Use of mild topical corticosteroids for acute flares.

Urticaria

A transient, immunologically mediated skin reaction presenting as raised, itchy welts or hives. It can be triggered by allergens,

medications, or physical factors such as heat or cold.
Key Features:
Rapid appearance of wheels that are pale at the center with erythematous borders.
Lesions resolve within hours to days but may recur.
Angioedema may accompany urticaria in severe cases, particularly around the face and airways.
Management:
Elimination of known triggers.
Antihistamines (e.g., loratadine or cetirizine) to control symptoms.
Emergency care for angioedema or anaphylaxis.

Pellagra
A nutritional deficiency disease caused by inadequate intake of niacin (vitamin B3) or its precursor, tryptophan. Common in populations with a diet heavily reliant on corn or maize.
Key Features:
Dermatitis: Symmetrical, well-defined, hyperpigmented, scaly patches, primarily in sun-exposed areas.
Other Symptoms: Diarrhea, dementia, and eventual death if

untreated (the "3 Ds" of pellagra).
Skin lesions may worsen with sun exposure and resemble a photosensitivity reaction.
Management:
Niacin supplementation, either orally or intravenously for severe cases.
Addressing underlying causes, such as malnutrition or malabsorption.
By recognizing these varied skin disorders and implementing appropriate treatment strategies, clinicians can effectively address both the physical and underlying causes of these conditions.

Chapter 5
Eye diseases

This chapter addresses a spectrum of significant eye diseases, focusing on their clinical features, underlying causes, and management approaches:
Xerophthalmia (Vitamin A Deficiency): Highlights the role of vitamin A deficiency in progressive eye damage, emphasizing prevention through supplementation and dietary improvements.

Conjunctivitis: Reviews the causes and presentation of conjunctival inflammation, differentiating between bacterial, viral, and allergic forms for tailored treatment.

Neonatal Conjunctivitis: Discusses its infectious origins and the critical need for prompt intervention to prevent complications such as corneal damage.

Viral Epidemic Keratoconjunctivitis: Explores this highly contagious eye condition caused by adenovirus, focusing on supportive care and infection control measures.

Trachoma: Examines this chronic infectious disease caused by Chlamydia trachomatis, highlighting its prevention and treatment to avert blindness.

Periorbital and Orbital Cellulitis: Differentiates between superficial and deep infections around the eye, stressing early diagnosis and antibiotic therapy to prevent complications.

Other Pathologies: Includes discussions on less common but notable conditions affecting eye health.

Onchocerciasis (River Blindness): Reviews this parasitic disease caused by Onchocerca volvulus, with emphasis on its transmission, diagnosis, and ivermectin treatment.

Loiasis: Discusses the clinical presentation of this filarial infection and its management, including antiparasitic therapy.

Pterygium: Details the growth of fibrovascular tissue over the cornea, focusing on prevention and surgical intervention in severe cases.

Cataract: Explores the leading cause of reversible blindness globally, emphasizing surgical correction and advancements in lens replacement techniques.

Xerophthalmia (Vitamin A Deficiency)

Xerophthalmia encompasses all ocular manifestations caused by vitamin A deficiency. Without intervention, it can lead to irreversible blindness. The condition primarily affects malnourished children, particularly those with measles, and pregnant women in endemic areas.

Clinical Features:
Hemeralopia (Night Blindness): Early symptom where children struggle to see in dim light, often bumping into objects.
Conjunctival Xerosis: Dry, thick, and wrinkled bulbar conjunctiva.
Bitot's Spots: Grayish foamy patches on the conjunctiva, although not always present.
Corneal Xerosis: Dry and dull corneal surface.
Keratomalacia: Advanced stage involving corneal softening, perforation, and blindness.
Treatment:
Early treatment can save vision, provided the pupil is spared, and corneal damage affects less than one-third of the surface.
Administer retinol (Vitamin A):
Children <6 months: 50,000 IU on Day 1, Day 2, and Day 8.
Children 6 months–1 year: 100,000 IU on the same schedule.
Children ≥1 year and adults: 200,000 IU following the same protocol.
For pregnant women, dosage adjustments are made to minimize teratogenic risks.
Prevention:

Routine vitamin A supplementation for children and postpartum women in endemic areas reduces incidence. Adequate dosing prevents toxic side effects like raised intracranial pressure.

Conjunctivitis

Conjunctivitis, an inflammation of the conjunctiva, arises from bacterial, viral, allergic, or irritative causes. Poor hygiene and untreated cases can lead to corneal involvement.

Clinical Features:

Bacterial: Purulent discharge, eyelids sticking together, usually unilateral at onset.

Viral: Watery discharge, no itching.

Allergic: Intense itching, eyelid swelling, excessive tearing.

Treatment:

Bacterial Conjunctivitis: Clean eyes with saline and apply tetracycline eye ointment twice daily for seven days.

Viral Conjunctivitis: Maintain hygiene and avoid corticosteroid drops.

Allergic Conjunctivitis: Use antihistamines for short-term relief.

Neonatal Conjunctivitis

This medical emergency is caused by Neisseria gonorrhoeae or Chlamydia trachomatis from maternal infections during delivery. Untreated, it risks corneal damage and visual impairment.

Clinical Features:
Purulent discharge within the first 28 days of life.

Treatment:
Systemic antibiotics:
Ceftriaxone IM: 50 mg/kg single dose (maximum 125 mg).
Azithromycin PO: 20 mg/kg daily for three days.
Cleanse eyes with sterile solutions regularly.
Treat maternal and partner infections simultaneously.

Prevention:
Apply 1% tetracycline eye ointment to neonates within one hour of birth. Monitor for adverse effects like pyloric stenosis associated with macrolides.

References

1. Lund, M., et al. "Use of Macrolides in Mother and Child and Risk of Infantile Hypertrophic Pyloric Stenosis:

Nationwide Cohort Study." BMJ, vol. 348, 2014, g1908.
2. Murchison, L., et al. "Post-Natal Erythromycin Exposure and Risk of Infantile Hypertrophic Pyloric Stenosis: A Systematic Review and Meta-Analysis." Pediatric Surgery International, vol. 32, no. 12, 2016, pp. 1147-1152.
3. Almaramhy, H. H., et al. "The Association of Prenatal and Postnatal Macrolide Exposure with Subsequent Development of Infantile Hypertrophic Pyloric Stenosis: A Systematic Review and Meta-Analysis." Italian Journal of Pediatrics, vol. 45, no. 1, 2019, Article 20.

Viral Epidemic Keratoconjunctivitis
Corneal and Conjunctival Lesions:
Viral keratoconjunctivitis should be treated as a typical viral conjunctivitis. Referral to an ophthalmologist is recommended when possible. During episodes of photophobia, the eye should be protected using a compress. The compress should be removed as soon as the photophobia subsides. In cases where

preventive care is needed, administering vitamin A is advisable.

Trachoma

Trachoma is a highly contagious infection of the cornea and conjunctiva caused by Chlamydia trachomatis. This disease is predominantly found in underdeveloped rural regions in Africa, Asia, the Middle East, and parts of Central and South America.

The infection often begins in early childhood through direct or indirect contact, such as unwashed hands, contaminated towels, or flies. In the absence of proper hygiene and effective treatment, repeated infections lead to persistent inflammation. This chronic condition causes scarring on the upper tarsal conjunctiva, resulting in ingrown eyelashes (trichiasis), which can cause corneal damage and, ultimately, irreversible blindness in adulthood.

The World Health Organization (WHO) divides trachoma into five stages, and early diagnosis and treatment are crucial in preventing the progression to trichiasis and its complications.

Clinical Features:

The stages of trachoma may overlap, and the disease can progress through several distinct phases:

1. Stage 1: Trachomatous Inflammation - Follicular (TF)

This stage is characterized by the presence of five or more follicles on the upper tarsal conjunctiva. The follicles appear as pale, whitish, gray, or yellow elevations, contrasting with the surrounding conjunctiva.

2. Stage 2: Trachomatous Inflammation - Intense (TI)

The upper tarsal conjunctiva appears red, rough, and thickened. Blood vessels are obscured by diffuse inflammatory infiltration or follicles.

3. Stage 3: Trachomatous Scarring (TS)

As the inflammation subsides, the follicles fade, leaving behind white scars in the tarsal conjunctiva.

4. Stage 4: Trachomatous Trichiasis (TT)

Due to scarring, the eyelid margin, particularly the upper lid, turns inward (entropion). This causes the eyelashes to rub against the cornea, resulting in ulcerations and chronic inflammation.

5. Stage 5: Corneal Opacity (CO)
As the disease progresses, the cornea becomes increasingly opaque, leading to visual impairment and blindness.

Treatment:

Stages 1 and 2:
Frequent cleaning of the eyes and face is crucial, and antibiotic therapy is recommended. The preferred treatment is a single oral dose of azithromycin:
Children: 20 mg/kg
Adults: 1 g
If azithromycin is not available or fails, alternatives include:
1% tetracycline eye ointment: applied twice daily for 6 weeks.
Erythromycin: 20 mg/kg (maximum 1 g) twice daily for 14 days.

Stage 3:
No specific treatment is required at this stage, as the scarring is irreversible.

Stage 4:

Surgical intervention is necessary. If surgery is not immediately available, a temporary palliative measure is to tape the ingrowing eyelashes to the eyelid. This procedure can help protect the cornea and, in some cases, may result in permanent correction of trichiasis within a few months. The method involves using a thin strip of tape to affix the eyelashes to the eyelid, ensuring that the eyelid can still open and close. The tape should be replaced weekly for up to 3 months.

Stage 5:

No effective treatment is available for corneal opacity at this stage, as the damage to the cornea is usually irreversible.

Prevention:

Regular cleaning of the eyes, face, and hands with clean water helps reduce transmission and the risk of secondary bacterial infections. It is important to note that epilation (plucking) of ingrown eyelashes is not recommended, as it only offers temporary relief, and regrowing eyelashes may cause more damage to the cornea.

References

1. Solomon, A. W., et al. "The Simplified Trachoma Grading System, Amended." Bulletin of the World Health Organization, vol. 98, no. 10, 2020, pp. 698-705.
2. Thylefors, B., et al. "A Simple System for the Assessment of Trachoma and Its Complications." Bulletin of the World Health Organization, vol. 65, no. 4, 1987, pp. 477-483.
3. Evans, J. R., et al. "Antibiotics for Trachoma." Cochrane Database of Systematic Reviews, 2019, CD001860.

Periorbital and Orbital Cellulitis: Periorbital cellulitis is a common and typically mild bacterial infection affecting the eyelids, often following trauma such as insect bites or abrasions. In contrast, orbital cellulitis is a more severe infection involving the structures within the eye socket, including the fat and ocular muscles. This condition can lead to complications like vision loss or brain abscesses, and it is commonly a

complication of sinusitis, particularly ethmoid sinusitis.
Both conditions are more frequently observed in children than adults. The primary pathogens responsible for both periorbital and orbital cellulitis include Staphylococcus aureus, Streptococcus pneumoniae, and other streptococci, as well as Haemophilus influenzae type b (Hib), particularly in regions with low Hib vaccination rates.

Clinical Features:
Common symptoms for both conditions:
Acute eyelid erythema and swelling.
If caused by Haemophilus influenzae, the swelling may have a violaceous (purple) hue.
Symptoms unique to orbital cellulitis:
Pain upon eye movement.
Ophthalmoplegia (impaired eye movement) often accompanied by diplopia (double vision).
Proptosis (eye bulging out of the socket).
High fever and other systemic signs of infection.
Treatment Guidelines:

1. Hospitalization is necessary for:
Orbital cellulitis.
Neonates (children under 3 months) and critically ill patients.
Cases with local complications, those with chronic conditions, or the elderly.
Situations where there is concern about patient compliance with outpatient treatment.
2. Outpatient Treatment:
Oral antibiotics are prescribed for 7-10 days:
Cefalexin (oral):
Neonates (0-7 days): 25 mg/kg twice daily.
Neonates (8 days to 1 month): 25 mg/kg three times daily.
Children >1 month: 25 mg/kg twice daily (max. 2 g daily).
Children ≥40 kg and adults: 1 g twice daily.
Amoxicillin/clavulanic acid (co-amoxiclav) (oral):
Children <40 kg: 50 mg/kg twice daily.
Children ≥40 kg and adults:
Ratio 8:1: 3000 mg daily (two 500/62.5 mg tablets three times daily).

Ratio 7:1: 2625 mg daily (one 875/125 mg tablet three times daily).
3. Inpatient Treatment:
Ceftriaxone (IV):
Children: Start with 100 mg/kg on the first day, then 50 mg/kg twice daily.
Adults: 1-2 g once daily.
Cloxacillin (IV):
Neonates (0-7 days, < 2 kg): 50 mg/kg every 12 hours.
Neonates (0-7 days, ≥ 2 kg): 50 mg/kg every 8 hours.
Neonates (8 days to 1 month, < 2 kg): 50 mg/kg every 8 hours.
Neonates (8 days to 1 month, ≥ 2 kg): 50 mg/kg every 6 hours.
Children >1 month: 25-50 mg/kg every 6 hours (max. 8 g daily).
Adults ≥40 kg: 2 g every 6 hours.
4. If there is no clinical improvement after 48 hours, suspect methicillin-resistant S. aureus (MRSA):
Switch cloxacillin to clindamycin (IV):
Neonates (0-7 days, < 2 kg): 5 mg/kg every 12 hours.
Neonates (0-7 days, ≥ 2 kg): 5 mg/kg every 8 hours.
Neonates (8 days to 1 month, < 2 kg): 5 mg/kg every 8 hours.

Neonates (8 days to 1 month, ≥ 2 kg): 10 mg/kg every 8 hours.
Children >1 month: 10 mg/kg every 8 hours (max. 1800 mg daily).
Adults: 600 mg every 8 hours.
5. After 5 days of IV antibiotics, switch to oral antibiotics for completion of a 7-10 day course, depending on the patient's clinical response.
6. Alternative treatments for penicillin-allergic patients:
Clindamycin (oral or IV) can be used for 7-10 days:
Children (oral): 10 mg/kg three times daily.
Adults (oral): 600 mg three times daily.
Footnotes for Special Considerations:
Critically ill children: These patients may present with weak crying, difficulty waking up, abnormal eye movement, or signs of cyanosis and hypotonia.
For patients with penicillin allergy, the recommended regimen involves clindamycin.
Reconstitution and administration of IV antibiotics should follow proper dilution

protocols to ensure efficacy and safety.
Other Pathologies:
1. Onchocerciasis: A parasitic infection caused by Onchocerca volvulus, transmitted through the bite of infected blackflies. It can lead to skin and eye issues, including blindness (river blindness).
2. Loiasis: Caused by Loa loa worms, transmitted by deer flies. It results in symptoms like swelling of the skin and can affect the eyes, causing visual disturbances.
3. Pterygium: A benign growth of tissue on the conjunctiva that may extend to the cornea, often caused by prolonged exposure to UV light. It can lead to irritation or vision impairment.
4. Cataract: A clouding of the eye's lens that impairs vision, commonly associated with aging, but also linked to trauma, genetics, or other health conditions like diabetes.
Onchocerciasis (River Blindness):
Onchocerciasis is a parasitic infection caused by Onchocerca volvulus, with ocular lesions

resulting from the invasion of the eye by microfilariae. These lesions can lead to irreversible blindness if left untreated. Ocular manifestations are always accompanied by skin lesions, such as pruritus, which is discussed in Chapter 6 on Onchocerciasis. The infection commonly affects the cornea, iris, and posterior segment of the eye.

Clinical Features:
Pruritus (itching)
Hemeralopia (night blindness)
Decreased visual acuity
Narrowing of the visual field
Microfilariae observed in the visual field, often described by patients as "little wiggling worms"
Corneal lesions: Punctate keratitis progressing to sclerosing keratitis
Iris involvement: Iridocyclitis
Posterior segment involvement: Chorioretinopathy and optic atrophy

Management and Treatment:
Early intervention is critical. Ivermectin is the drug of choice for treatment, as it can improve anterior segment lesions, such as

sclerosing keratitis and iridocyclitis, and may improve visual acuity. However, severe lesions like chorioretinal damage and optic atrophy may continue to progress despite treatment. Ocular management may involve supportive care for visual impairments, while systemic ivermectin helps control the infection and prevent further ocular damage. Long-term management focuses on controlling the infection to prevent progression of blindness.

Loiasis:

Loiasis, caused by Loa loa, is characterized by the migration of adult worms under the conjunctiva. The worms are usually visible as mobile, white, thread-like structures measuring between 4 to 7 cm in length. This condition primarily causes discomfort in the form of itching and other ocular symptoms.

Clinical Features:

Migration of the adult worm under the palpebral or bulbar conjunctiva, visible as a mobile, white filiform worm

Ocular pruritus (itching)

Lacrimation (tearing)

Photophobia (light sensitivity)
Eyelid edema
Management and Treatment:
The migration of the worm is usually brief and does not require extraction. It is important to avoid attempts at removing the worm or administering anesthetic drops, as these may cause further irritation or complications. Patients should be reassured that the condition is typically harmless and resolves on its own. If the worm is dead or calcified, surgical removal is unnecessary and ineffective. Treatment with diethylcarbamazine (DEC) may be used in certain cases to reduce microfilarial load and prevent further migration. Further management focuses on symptomatic relief and monitoring for any potential complications.

Pterygium:
Pterygium is a benign growth of fibrovascular tissue that extends from the conjunctiva onto the cornea. It is most commonly seen in individuals who have prolonged exposure to environmental irritants such as wind, dust, or dry, arid climates.

Pterygium typically does not resolve spontaneously and may progress over time, affecting vision if it reaches the central cornea.
Clinical Features:
A triangular growth of vascular tissue extending from the conjunctiva onto the cornea
Initially benign and asymptomatic, with no immediate effect on vision
In progressive pterygium, the growth becomes vascularized, red, and inflamed, potentially obstructing the pupil and impairing vision
Irritation and discomfort due to the growth of tissue over the cornea
May cause visual impairment if it covers the central cornea or if it induces astigmatism
Management and Treatment:
Benign pterygium: When the growth does not extend to the pupil and causes minimal discomfort, no treatment is necessary. Regular monitoring is recommended to ensure it does not progress.
Progressive pterygium: For more symptomatic or visually

impairing growths, initial treatment includes lubricating eye drops (sterile saline or 0.9% sodium chloride) to reduce irritation. Surgical excision is the treatment of choice if the pterygium progresses to cover the pupil or significantly affects vision. Post-surgery, patients may be prescribed anti-inflammatory medications to prevent recurrence, as pterygium has a tendency to return.

Cataract:

A cataract is the clouding of the lens of the eye, leading to a gradual loss of visual clarity. It is a common condition, especially in tropical regions, and can occur at younger ages compared to Western countries. Cataracts are typically progressive, leading to eventual blindness if both eyes are affected.

Clinical Features:

Gradual loss of visual acuity, often starting with blurred vision or difficulty seeing at night

Glare and halos around lights, especially at night

Double vision or ghosting of images

Cloudy or opaque appearance of the lens, visible upon examination

Management and Treatment:
The primary treatment for cataracts is surgical intervention. During cataract surgery, the cloudy lens is removed and typically replaced with an intraocular lens (IOL) to restore vision. The surgery is highly successful, with most patients regaining significant vision improvement. Postoperative care involves the use of antibiotics and anti-inflammatory drops to prevent infection and manage inflammation. In non-surgical cases, vision can be managed with stronger corrective lenses or glasses, but surgery is ultimately required for significant visual impairment.

Chapter 6
Parasitic Diseases

This chapter covers a range of parasitic infections, including:

Malaria: A mosquito-borne disease caused by Plasmodium species, leading to fever, chills, and potentially severe complications.

Human African Trypanosomiasis (Sleeping Sickness): Caused by Trypanosoma species, transmitted by tsetse flies, leading to neurological symptoms and sleep disturbances.
American Trypanosomiasis (Chagas Disease): Caused by Trypanosoma cruzi, transmitted by triatomine bugs, affecting the heart and digestive system.
Leishmaniasis: A group of diseases caused by Leishmania parasites, transmitted by sandflies, with cutaneous, mucocutaneous, and visceral forms.
Intestinal Protozoan Infections (Parasitic Diarrhea): Infections from protozoa like Entamoeba, causing gastrointestinal symptoms such as diarrhea and abdominal pain.
Flukes: Parasitic flatworms, including liver, lung, and blood flukes, causing diseases like schistosomiasis and fascioliasis.
Schistosomiasis: A disease caused by Schistosoma species, leading to liver, intestine, or urinary tract damage.

Cestodes (Tapeworms): Parasitic flatworms that infect the intestines, often causing nutritional deficiencies and abdominal discomfort.
Nematode Infections: Infections from roundworms, including diseases like ascariasis, trichuriasis, and strongyloidiasis.
Filariasis: A parasitic infection caused by filarial worms, leading to lymphatic damage and conditions such as elephantiasis.
Onchocerciasis (River Blindness): Caused by Onchocerca volvulus, transmitted by blackflies, leading to skin and eye lesions, and eventual blindness.
Loiasis: Caused by Loa loa, characterized by migrating adult worms under the skin and conjunctiva.
Lymphatic Filariasis (LF): Caused by filarial worms, affecting the lymphatic system, leading to swelling and elephantiasis.
Malaria: A Detailed Overview
Malaria is a parasitic infection caused by protozoa from the Plasmodium genus, primarily transmitted to humans through

the bite of an infected Anopheles mosquito. Transmission can also occur via transfusion of infected blood or through transplacental routes.

Five Plasmodium species are responsible for malaria in humans:

P. falciparum
P.
P. ovale
P. malariae
P.

While all these species can cause uncomplicated malaria, P. falciparum is most commonly associated with severe malaria, which may lead to death within hours if untreated. Although less common, severe malaria can also be caused by P. and P. .

Clinical Features of Malaria

1. Uncomplicated Malaria:

Symptoms typically include fever, chills, sweating, headache, muscle aches, malaise, anorexia, and nausea.

In children, gastrointestinal symptoms such as abdominal pain, diarrhea, and vomiting are common.

Mild to moderate anemia is frequently observed, especially in children and pregnant women.
2. Severe Malaria:
Characterized by the presence of serious complications such as:
Impaired consciousness or coma
Seizures (more than two episodes within 24 hours)
Prostration (extreme weakness, inability to sit or drink in children)
Respiratory distress (rapid, labored breathing or slow, deep breathing)
Shock (cold extremities, weak or absent pulse, delayed capillary refill, cyanosis)
Jaundice (yellow discoloration of mucosal surfaces)
Hemoglobinuria (dark red urine)
Abnormal bleeding (petechiae, gum bleeding, blood in stools)
Acute renal failure (oliguria despite adequate hydration)
Diagnosis of Malaria
Parasitological Diagnosis: Malaria diagnosis should be confirmed with parasitological tests. However, treatment should not be delayed if diagnostic tests are unavailable.

1. Microscopy: Thin and thick blood films are used to detect the presence of parasites, identify species, and quantify parasitemia. However, severe malaria may result in sequestration of parasitized red blood cells in peripheral capillaries, leading to negative results despite infection.
2. Rapid Diagnostic Tests (RDTs): These tests detect parasite antigens and provide a qualitative result (positive or negative). However, they may remain positive for several days to weeks, even after parasite elimination.
3. Additional Laboratory Examinations:
Hemoglobin Levels: To assess anemia, routinely measured in all patients with clinical anemia or severe malaria.
Blood Glucose Levels: Monitoring is crucial to detect hypoglycemia, especially in severe malaria cases or patients with malnutrition.
Treatment of Malaria
1. Uncomplicated Malaria:
For P. , P. ovale, P. malariae, and P. knowlesi, chloroquine (CQ) is

typically administered orally in the following doses:
Day 1: 10 mg base/kg
Day 2: 10 mg base/kg
Day 3: 5 mg base/kg
P. may show resistance to chloroquine in some regions. In such cases or where resistance is high, artemisinin-based combination therapy (ACT) should be used.
*Relapse prevention for P. and P. ovale involves a 14-day course of primaquine after the initial treatment to eliminate dormant liver-stage parasites. However, primaquine is contraindicated in individuals with G6PD deficiency.

2. Uncomplicated P. falciparum Malaria:
The preferred treatment is ACT, administered orally for 3 days. The choice of ACT depends on the local resistance patterns. If first-line ACT is unavailable or ineffective, an alternative ACT should be used.
In areas with low malaria transmission, primaquine is given as a single dose to reduce transmission risk.

3. Severe Malaria:

Hospitalization is required for severe malaria. Antimalarial treatment is administered parenterally, with artesunate being the drug of choice. If artesunate is unavailable, artemether may be used. The dosages are:
Children < 20 kg: 3 mg/kg/dose
Adults & children ≥ 20 kg: 2.4 mg/kg/dose
Parenteral treatment should be continued for at least 24 hours before switching to oral therapy if the patient can tolerate it.
Alternative Treatments:
Quinine can be used in some national protocols for malaria with shock when artesunate is unavailable. Quinine should be given intravenously or intramuscularly, with the dosing adjusted based on body weight.
Pre-Referral Treatment: Before transferring a patient, the first dose of artesunate (or artemether if artesunate is unavailable) should be administered.
4. Symptomatic Treatment:
Fever: Use paracetamol to manage high fever.

Severe Anemia: Blood transfusion may be necessary if anemia is significant.

Hypoglycemia: Patients should be monitored and treated with glucose if necessary.

5. Managing Complications:

Hydration: Patients should receive adequate hydration to prevent dehydration and avoid fluid overload, which can lead to pulmonary edema.

Respiratory Distress: In case of pulmonary edema, reduce IV infusion rates, administer oxygen, and consider furosemide if necessary.

Seizures: Treat according to standard protocols, including addressing possible hypoglycemia or fever.

Acute Renal Failure: In severe cases, urinary catheterization and close monitoring of fluid balance are crucial.

Conclusion

Malaria remains a significant global health challenge. Early detection and appropriate treatment are essential to prevent complications and death. Antimalarial therapy is effective in treating uncomplicated malaria, while severe malaria requires immediate hospitalization and aggressive treatment. Supportive care for complications, including hydration, fever management, and monitoring for organ failure, is critical for improving outcomes.

References

1. World Health Organization (WHO). Malaria Treatment Guidelines, 3rd edition. WHO, 2015. Available at: https://apps.who.int/iris/handle/10665/162441

2. World Health Organization (WHO). Compendium of WHO Malaria Guidance: Prevention, Diagnosis, Treatment, Surveillance, and Elimination. WHO, 2019. Available at: https://apps.who.int/iris/handle/10665/312082

3. World Health Organization (WHO). Policy Brief on Single-Dose Primaquine as a Gametocytocide in Plasmodium falciparum Malaria. WHO, 2015. Available at: https://www.who.int/malaria/publications/atoz/who_htm_gmp_2015.1.pdf?ua=1

4. World Health Organization (WHO). Policy Recommendation on Seasonal Malaria Chemoprevention (SMC) for Plasmodium falciparum Malaria Control in Highly Seasonal Transmission Areas of the Sahel Sub-region in Africa. WHO, 2012.

Human African Trypanosomiasis (HAT) (Sleeping Sickness)

Human African Trypanosomiasis (HAT) is a zoonotic disease caused by protozoan parasites of the Trypanosoma genus. The disease is primarily transmitted to humans through the bite of the tsetse fly (Glossina), although transmission via contaminated blood transfusions and from mother to child (transplacental) is also possible. HAT is endemic in sub-Saharan Africa and manifests in two distinct forms: Trypanosoma brucei gambiense (HAT), prevalent in western and central Africa, and Trypanosoma (HAT), found in eastern and southern Africa.

Clinical Presentation

Upon inoculation, a local reaction known as a trypanosomal change may develop. This occurs in around 50% of T. b. cases but rarely in T. b. infections.

Stages of Disease:

HAT: The disease progresses more slowly, with a prolonged incubation period (often years). Initial symptoms are subtle, but as the disease progresses, it leads to neurological symptoms like sleep disturbances, psychiatric changes, and motor dysfunction.

HAT: The disease progresses rapidly, often within weeks. Acute symptoms include fever, myalgia, and lymphadenopathy, and the disease can progress to myocarditis and death within 3 to 6 months without treatment.

Differentiating between and forms can be challenging due to the potential overlap in symptom presentation, such as acute infections or chronic cases.

Laboratory Findings:

The disease progresses in two stages:

1. Hemolymphatic Stage (Stage I): Parasites disseminate via the bloodstream and lymphatic system, leading to intermittent fever, joint pain, lymphadenopathy (particularly

cervical), hepatosplenomegaly, and cutaneous signs like facial edema and pruritus.
2. Meningoencephalitis Stage (Stage II): The parasite invades the central nervous system, leading to neurological symptoms such as sensory disturbances, psychiatric changes, sleep cycle disruptions, motor impairment (paralysis, seizures), and endocrine issues like amenorrhea and impotence. Without treatment, patients experience cachexia, lethargy, coma, and death.

Diagnosis:
Diagnosis involves a multi-step approach, including:
Screening (for T. b.): The Card Agglutination Test for Trypanosomiasis (CATT) detects antibodies in the blood or serum.
Diagnostic Confirmation: Trypanosomes are identified through lymph node aspirates, blood samples, or specialized techniques such as capillary tube centrifugation (Woo test) or mini-anion exchange centrifugation (mAEC).
Stage Determination: A lumbar puncture is conducted to analyze

cerebrospinal fluid (CSF). In the hemolymphatic stage, trypanosomes are absent, and white blood cell counts are ≤5 cells/mm^3. In the meningoencephalitis stage, trypanosomes are present, or the CSF white cell count exceeds 5 cells/mm^3.

Treatment:
Treatment varies depending on the disease stage:

Hemolymphatic Stage (Stage I)
HAT: Pentamidine is administered intramuscularly (IM) at 4 mg/kg/day for 7 to 10 days. Patients should be monitored for hypoglycemia and hypotension.
HAT: Suramin is given intravenously (IV) in a slow infusion, starting with a test dose followed by a maintenance dose over several weeks.

Meningoencephalitis Stage (Stage II)
Before administering trypanocides, supportive treatments such as rehydration and treatment of concurrent infections are prioritized. However, trypanocidal treatment

should not be delayed for more than 10 days.

First-line treatment: Nifurtimox-eflornithine combination therapy (NEXT) is the preferred regimen. Nifurtimox is given orally (5 mg/kg 3 times daily), combined with eflornithine (200 mg/kg IV infusion every 12 hours for 7 days).

Second-line treatment: In cases of relapse, melarsoprol (slow IV infusion) is used, despite its high toxicity. It can cause reactive encephalopathy, which may lead to coma or prolonged seizures.

Special Considerations in Pregnant Women: All trypanocidal drugs pose potential risks to both the mother and fetus. For pregnant women:

Hemolymphatic Stage: Pentamidine is used for T. b. infections, and suramin for T. b.

Meningoencephalitis Stage: If the mother's condition is life-threatening, NEXT or eflornithine should not be deferred. If not life-threatening, pentamidine or suramin may be used until after delivery, when more aggressive treatments can be started.

Prevention:

Prevention of HAT relies on individual protection against tsetse fly bites, which includes wearing long sleeves and trousers, using insect repellents, and avoiding tsetse fly habitats. Mass screening and treatment are critical for controlling T. b. infections, while vector control strategies such as tsetse fly traps or insecticides help manage T. b. . Cattle, which can harbor T. b. , may also need to be treated.

American Trypanosomiasis (Chagas Disease)

disease, caused by the protozoan Trypanosoma , is transmitted primarily by triatomine bugs. Transmission can occur through the bug's feces, which contaminate breaks in the skin or mucous membranes, but it can also be spread via contaminated blood transfusions, congenital transmission, or consumption of contaminated food and water. disease is predominantly found in the Americas and is often underdiagnosed.

Clinical Features:

Acute Phase: This phase typically lasts for 4 to 6 weeks and can present with symptoms such as a red swelling at the site of infection (chagoma), unilateral periorbital swelling (Romaña's sign), fever, lymphadenopathy, hepatosplenomegaly, and occasionally myocarditis or meningoencephalitis.

Chronic Phase: Most individuals enter a long indeterminate phase where symptoms are absent, but up to 30% of cases progress to chronic complications. These include cardiac manifestations (such as arrhythmias, dilated cardiomyopathy), gastrointestinal issues (like megaesophagus and megacolon), and neurological problems. Immunosuppressed individuals are at higher risk for severe organ damage.

Diagnosis:

Acute Phase: The presence of T. can be detected in blood samples via direct microscopy or concentration techniques such as the microhematocrit method.

Chronic Phase: Diagnosis is confirmed through serologic tests that detect antibodies against T. , using methods like ELISA or indirect immunofluorescence. In some cases, two serological tests are required for confirmation.

Treatment:

Aetiological Treatment: Benznidazole and nifurtimox are the primary treatments. However, treatment is most effective during the acute phase or early chronic phase. For patients with severe cardiac or digestive complications, treatment may not be recommended.

Benznidazole: Administered orally (5–8 mg/kg daily for 60 days for children; 5–7 mg/kg for adults).

Nifurtimox: Administered orally (15–20 mg/kg daily for children, 8–10 mg/kg for adults) for 90 days.

Both medications are contraindicated during pregnancy and breastfeeding, and patients must be monitored closely due to common side effects, including gastrointestinal disturbances and central nervous system effects.

Prevention:

Preventative measures focus on reducing exposure to triatomine bugs, improving housing conditions, and screening blood donors in endemic areas to prevent transmission via blood transfusions.

References

1. Pan American Health Organization. (2019). Guidelines for the diagnosis and treatment of Chagas disease. Washington, D.C. Retrieved from http://iris.paho.org/xmlui/bitstream/handle/123456789/49653/9789275120439_eng.pdf?sequence=6&isAllowed=y

2. Rassi, A., & Marin-Neto, J. (2010). Seminar: Chagas disease. The Lancet, 375(9723), 1388-1402. https://doi.org/10.1016/S0140-6736(10)60061-X

3. Centers for Disease Control and Prevention. (2020). Parasites - American Trypanosomiasis. Retrieved February 17, 2020, from https://www.cdc.gov/parasites/chagas/

4. World Health Organization. (1995). WHO Model Prescribing Information: Drugs Used in Parasitic Diseases - Second Edition. Geneva. Retrieved May 6, 2020, from

https://apps.who.int/iris/handle/10665/41765

Leishmaniasis Overview

Leishmaniasis refers to a group of parasitic diseases caused by Leishmania species, transmitted by the bite of infected sandflies. Over 20 different species can cause leishmaniasis in humans.

Clinical Presentation

1. Cutaneous and Mucocutaneous Leishmaniasis

Cutaneous leishmaniasis commonly presents with a single or multiple skin lesions, typically beginning as erythematous papules at the site of a sandfly bite. These lesions can develop into nodules and then ulcers, which may become crusted. Though usually painless, these ulcers can become painful if infected by bacteria or fungi.

Mucocutaneous leishmaniasis, which is more common in Latin America and occasionally in Africa, results when lesions spread to mucosal areas (mouth, nose, or eyes), often leading to severe disfigurement.

2. Visceral Leishmaniasis (Kala-azar)

Visceral leishmaniasis is a systemic infection that can result in severe consequences, including pancytopenia (a deficiency of red blood cells, white blood cells, and platelets), immunosuppression, and, if untreated, death.

3. Post-Kala-Azar Dermal Leishmaniasis (PKDL)

Post-kala-azar dermal leishmaniasis can appear after a patient appears to recover from visceral leishmaniasis, presenting as a rash that may be macular, nodular, or papular, especially on the face. This condition can be disfiguring.

Laboratory Diagnosis

Cutaneous and Mucocutaneous Leishmaniasis: Diagnosis is typically based on the identification of Leishmania parasites in tissue biopsy samples, usually taken from the ulcer edges.

Visceral Leishmaniasis: Diagnosis involves parasitological techniques like the identification of Leishmania parasites in splenic, bone marrow, or lymph node biopsies. The most sensitive diagnostic method is splenic aspiration, though it carries a risk of severe bleeding. Serological tests like the rK39 dipstick and direct agglutination test (DAT) can be used in suspected cases.

Clinical Features of Visceral Leishmaniasis

Symptoms include prolonged fever (lasting over two weeks), splenomegaly (enlarged spleen), and weight loss. Additional signs may include anemia, diarrhea, epistaxis (nosebleeds), lymphadenopathy, and moderate hepatomegaly.

Immunosuppression can increase susceptibility to secondary infections like pneumonia, tuberculosis, and bacterial diarrhea.

Treatment Options

Cutaneous Leishmaniasis

Local treatment is recommended for lesions that are persistent, disfiguring, or ulcerating. First-line treatment involves pentavalent antimonial drugs like sodium stibogluconate or meglumine antimoniate, which are injected directly into the lesion. Treatment should be repeated every 3–7 days for 2–4 weeks.

In severe cases, systemic treatment with intramuscular pentavalent antimonials (20 mg/kg daily for 10–20 days) is needed.

Miltefosine, a systemic oral drug, can be effective for many forms of cutaneous leishmaniasis.

Antibiotics are prescribed for secondary infections like streptococcal or staphylococcal infections of the ulcers.

Visceral Leishmaniasis

For patients with visceral leishmaniasis, it is crucial to provide hydration, nutritional support, and treatment of co-infections (e.g., malaria, dysentery). If relapse occurs or treatment fails, HIV or tuberculosis should be considered.

First-line treatment involves pentavalent antimonials (20 mg/kg daily for 17 days) in combination with paromomycin (15 mg/kg daily for 17 days).

For patients with severe disease or for those with comorbid conditions like HIV, liposomal amphotericin B (3–5 mg/kg daily for 6–10 days) is recommended.

Post-Kala-Azar Dermal Leishmaniasis (PKDL)
Treatment for PKDL is indicated only for severe, disfiguring cases or persistent lesions lasting over 6 months. In East Africa, pentavalent antimonials combined with paromomycin or liposomal amphotericin B are commonly used. In South Asia, liposomal amphotericin B may be used with good results.

Prevention
Preventing leishmaniasis involves using insecticide-treated nets and controlling sandfly populations. Eliminating animal reservoirs (often dogs) also helps reduce transmission risks.

Intestinal Protozoan Infections
Common Protozoan Infections
Amoebiasis (caused by Entamoeba)
Giardiasis (caused by Giardia lamblia)
Cryptosporidiosis (caused by Cryptosporidium species)
Cyclosporiasis (caused by Cyclospora)
Isosporiasis (caused by Isospora belli)

These intestinal protozoa are transmitted via the fecal-oral route, typically through contaminated water or food. They cause diarrhea, which can range from mild to severe, especially in immunocompromised individuals.

Clinical Features

Diarrhea is the hallmark symptom, often accompanied by abdominal pain, distension, cramps, flatulence, nausea, and anorexia. In severe cases, particularly in immunocompromised individuals, diarrhea may be chronic or accompanied by malabsorption and significant weight loss.

Treatment

Giardiasis is treated with tinidazole (single oral dose) or metronidazole (for 3 days). Cryptosporidiosis in immunocompetent patients often resolves without treatment, but in immunocompromised patients, antiretroviral therapy (ART) should be considered.

Cyclosporiasis and Isosporiasis are treated with co-trimoxazole for 7 days.

Special Considerations for HIV Patients

In HIV-positive patients, intestinal protozoan infections may be opportunistic and require urgent treatment to prevent dehydration and further complications. Effective antiretroviral therapy (ART) should be initiated to boost immune function and reduce the risk of severe infection.

Fluke Infections

Lung Flukes (Paragonimus spp.)

Distribution: Predominantly found in Southeast Asia, China, parts of Africa, and South America.

Transmission: Ingestion of raw freshwater crustaceans.

Symptoms: Chronic productive cough and intermittent haemoptysis (coughing up rusty-brown sputum). The disease often mimics pulmonary tuberculosis.

Treatment: Praziquantel, administered orally (25 mg/kg three times daily for 2 days), is the treatment of choice.

Hepatobiliary Flukes (Fasciola hepatica and Fasciola)
Distribution: Worldwide in areas where livestock (e.g., sheep and cattle) are raised.
Transmission: Consumption of uncooked aquatic plants.
Symptoms: Early-stage symptoms may include fever, myalgia, and right upper quadrant pain. Once the flukes are established in the biliary tract, patients may present with obstructive jaundice and recurrent episodes of cholangitis.
Treatment: Triclabendazole is the drug of choice, given as a single oral dose (10 mg/kg). If the infection is severe, a second dose may be administered after 24 hours.

Footnotes
(a) For further details on the global distribution of schistosomiasis, refer to the World Health Organization's map: WHO Schistosomiasis Distribution Map.
(b) Praziquantel, the primary treatment for schistosomiasis, can be administered to pregnant women.

References

1. Medical Letter Treatment Guidelines, Vol. 11 (Suppl), Drugs for Parasitic Infections, 2013. Available at: Medical Letter on Parasitic Drugs [Accessed 25 May 2020].
2. Centers for Disease Control and Prevention (CDC). Schistosomiasis: Resources for Health Professionals, 2018. Available at: CDC Schistosomiasis Information [Accessed 25 May 2020].

Cestode Infections: Detailed Overview and Case-Based Analysis

Taeniasis (Taenia saginata and Taenia solium)

Taeniasis, caused by the tapeworm species Taenia saginata (beef tapeworm) and Taenia (pork tapeworm), is a globally prevalent infection, often presenting with minimal or no symptoms. When symptoms occur, they can include mild gastrointestinal disturbances, such as epigastric or abdominal pain, nausea, and diarrhea. Taenia eggs can be detected in stool samples or using the Scotch tape method to collect eggs from the perianal skin. Praziquantel is the treatment of choice, administered orally at a dosage of 5-10 mg/kg in a single dose for both children (aged 4 years and older) and adults.

Transmission and Prevention:
The primary mode of transmission is the ingestion of undercooked or raw beef (for T.) or pork (for T.). Preventive measures include cooking meat thoroughly and monitoring slaughterhouse practices to ensure meat safety.

Diphyllobothriasis
(Diphyllobothrium latum)
Diphyllobothriasis is caused by Diphyllobothrium , commonly found in temperate or cold freshwater lake regions. It often remains asymptomatic but can lead to mild gastrointestinal disturbances and, in cases of heavy infection, vitamin B12 deficiency and anemia. Neurological complications are rare but possible. Laboratory diagnosis is made by detecting eggs in stool samples. Treatment typically involves a single dose of praziquantel (5-10 mg/kg) for both children and adults (aged 4 years and older).

Transmission and Prevention:
The infection is transmitted through the consumption of raw or undercooked freshwater fish. Prevention includes thorough cooking of fish before consumption.

Hymenolepiasis (Hymenolepis nana)

Hymenolepis nana is a common cestode that causes hymenolepiasis, found worldwide. It is usually asymptomatic but can cause gastrointestinal disturbances, including epigastric pain, in cases of heavy infection. Diagnosis is confirmed by identifying eggs in stool samples. Praziquantel, at a dose of 15-25 mg/kg in a single dose for both children (aged 4 years and older) and adults, is the treatment of choice.

Transmission and Prevention:
Transmission occurs through the fecal-oral route or auto-infection. Preventive measures include proper hand hygiene, cutting nails, and ensuring proper sanitation and hygiene in communal settings such as water sources and latrines.

Cysticercosis (Taenia solium)
Cysticercosis, caused by Taenia, is a serious infection with a broad range of clinical manifestations. It can be asymptomatic, present as muscular pain, or cause neurological issues such as headaches, convulsions, and coma when the larvae affect the central nervous system. Subcutaneous nodules may also develop. Diagnosis typically shows hypereosinophilia in blood and cerebrospinal fluid samples. Neurocysticercosis and ocular cysticercosis require specialized care and may necessitate surgery. Anti-parasitic treatment should only be administered after proper diagnostic imaging (CT or MRI) to avoid exacerbating symptoms.
Transmission and Prevention:
The disease is transmitted by ingesting food contaminated with T. eggs or through auto-infection. Prevention involves treating T. carriers, practicing good hygiene, and thoroughly cooking meat from infected animals.
Hydatid Disease (Echinococcus)

Hydatid disease, caused by Echinococcus, is prevalent in South America, parts of Africa, and Western Europe. The cysts, primarily located in the liver (60% of cases) and lungs (30%), can cause significant complications, including biliary obstruction, anaphylactic shock upon cyst rupture, and jaundice. The treatment of choice is surgical excision, often supplemented with albendazole, especially in cases that are inoperable or post-surgery. Albendazole should be administered at 7.5 mg/kg for children over 2 years and adults weighing less than 60 kg, or 400 mg twice daily for those weighing more than 60 kg.

Transmission and Prevention: Transmission occurs through direct contact with infected dogs or indirectly through contaminated water or food. Preventive measures include avoiding contact with dogs, eliminating stray dogs, and monitoring slaughterhouse practices.

Nematode Infections

Ascariasis (Ascaris)

Ascariasis is a widespread infection caused by the roundworm Ascaris . During the larval migration phase, Loeffler's syndrome may occur, characterized by transient pulmonary symptoms (dry cough, wheezing) and mild fever. Once the adult worms mature in the intestines, symptoms include abdominal pain, distension, and, in severe cases, intestinal obstruction. Diagnosis is based on the detection of Ascaris eggs in stool samples. Treatment involves a single dose of albendazole (400 mg) or mebendazole (100 mg twice daily for 3 days).

Transmission and Prevention:
The infection is transmitted through the ingestion of Ascaris eggs, typically from contaminated food or water. Preventive measures include good hygiene and proper sanitation.

Trichuriasis (Trichuris trichiura)
Trichuris trichiura, the whipworm, causes trichuriasis, which may lead to abdominal pain, diarrhea, and, in severe cases, chronic bloody diarrhea,

tenesmus, and rectal prolapse. Diagnosis is confirmed by the presence of whipworm eggs in stool samples. Treatment includes albendazole (400 mg daily for 3 days) or mebendazole (administered in a similar regimen).

Transmission and Prevention:
Transmission is via ingestion of contaminated food or water, typically in tropical and subtropical regions. Preventive measures include ensuring proper sanitation and hand hygiene.

Hookworm Infections (Ancylostoma and Necator americanus)

Hookworm infections, caused by Ancylostoma and Necator americanus, are common in tropical and subtropical regions. The infection starts when larvae penetrate the skin, typically through contact with contaminated soil. Symptoms can include cutaneous reactions at the site of penetration and pulmonary symptoms during larval migration. Once the worms mature in the intestines, they cause mild abdominal pain and chronic blood loss, leading to anemia. Diagnosis is made by detecting hookworm eggs in stool samples. Treatment involves albendazole in a single dose, which is more effective than mebendazole.

Transmission and Prevention: Transmission occurs through skin contact with contaminated soil. Preventive measures include wearing shoes and ensuring proper sanitation.

Strongyloidiasis (Strongyloides stercoralis)

Strongyloidiasis is caused by Strongyloides, a nematode found in tropical and subtropical regions. It is transmitted through larval skin penetration and can cause cutaneous signs, such as erythema and pruritus, and pulmonary symptoms similar to ascariasis during larval migration. In chronic cases, the infection can lead to gastrointestinal symptoms and auto-infection. Hyperinfection, a severe form, can lead to systemic involvement, including CNS and heart. Diagnosis is through stool examination for larvae. The treatment of choice is ivermectin (200 micrograms/kg as a single

dose). In refractory cases, prolonged or multiple-dose regimens may be necessary.
Transmission and Prevention: Transmission occurs through skin contact with contaminated soil. Preventive measures include wearing protective footwear and practicing proper hygiene.

Enterobiasis (Pinworms)

Pinworm infection, caused by Enterobius, is common worldwide. It causes anal pruritus, particularly at night, and may lead to vulvovaginitis in girls. The diagnosis is usually made by collecting pinworm eggs from the perianal area using the Scotch tape method. Treatment involves a single dose of albendazole or mebendazole. A second dose is often recommended after 2 to 4 weeks.
Transmission and Prevention:
Pinworms are transmitted through the fecal-oral route or auto-infection. Preventive measures include handwashing and good personal hygiene.

Trichinellosis (Trichinella spp.)

Trichinellosis is caused by the ingestion of undercooked meat from animals infected with

Trichinella larvae, particularly pork, wart-hog, or bear meat. The disease progresses through an enteric phase, marked by self-limited diarrhea and abdominal pain, followed by a muscular phase characterized by high fever, muscular pain, and ocular edema. Diagnosis is confirmed through muscle biopsy or serology. Treatment involves albendazole, typically for 10 to 15 days.

Transmission and Prevention:
The disease is transmitted through the consumption of raw or undercooked meat containing Trichinella larvae. Preventive measures include thoroughly cooking meat to ensure safety.

Conclusion:
Cestode and nematode infections are globally prevalent and vary in severity based on the parasite involved and the individual's health status. Diagnosis often relies on stool samples or specialized tests, while treatment typically involves antiparasitic medications. Preventive measures, including proper hygiene and food safety

practices, are crucial in reducing transmission.

Footnote

(a) Sarcoptic scabies should be considered in the differential diagnosis (refer to Chapter 4 on Scabies).

(b) The elimination of Wolbachia reduces the lifespan and fertility of microfilariae, thereby decreasing microfilariae production.

(c) Ivermectin kills microfilariae and inhibits their production by adult worms, but it must be administered regularly, as it does not eliminate adult worms.

Loiasis:

Distribution:

Loiasis is found in regions where its vector, the Chrysops fly, is prevalent, primarily in forested or savannah areas of West and Central Africa. The geographic boundaries are West: Benin, East: Uganda, North: Sudan, and South: Angola.

Clinical Features:

Microfilaraemia (L. loa) typically ranges from 1,000 to 2,000 microfilariae per milliliter (mf/ml) of blood.

Symptoms include localized subcutaneous swellings (Calabar swellings), which are transient, painless, non-pitting, and often itchy, most frequently seen on the upper extremities and face.

Adult worm migration through the conjunctiva or subcutaneous tissue is pathognomonic of Loa loa infection. Subconjunctival migration of an adult worm is a key diagnostic feature.

Pruritus and migration of adult worms: This can present as a red, cord-like, moving linear lesion under the skin, which advances at a rate of approximately 1 cm/hour and resolves quickly without leaving a trace, typically after treatment with diethylcarbamazine (DEC).

Diagnosis:

Detection of microfilariae in peripheral blood via thick blood films (stained with Giemsa), ideally collected between 10 AM and 5 PM.

Quantification of microfilaraemia is critical to determine the intensity of infection and guide treatment. If positive, a differential diagnosis should be considered, especially where onchocerciasis is co-endemic.

Treatment:

1. Low Microfilaraemia (< 2,000 mf/ml):

A 28-day treatment with diethylcarbamazine (DEC) starting with a low dose of 6 mg (1/8 of a 50 mg tablet) twice daily, gradually increasing to 200 mg twice daily in adults (or 1.5 mg/kg twice daily for children).

If symptoms persist, a second round of treatment may be administered after 4 weeks.

If co-infection with Onchocerca volvulus is suspected or confirmed, ivermectin (150 µg/kg) is used to treat onchocerciasis and alleviate associated symptoms, such as pruritus and Calabar swellings. The ivermectin treatment can be repeated monthly or every 3 months.

2. Moderate Microfilaraemia (2,000–8,000 mf/ml):

Ivermectin (150 µg/kg single dose) is used to reduce microfilaraemia, followed by DEC when microfilariae count falls below 2,000 mf/ml.

Repeat ivermectin monthly if necessary.

3. High Microfilaraemia (8,000–30,000 mf/ml):

Ivermectin is used but requires careful supervision due to potential adverse effects, including functional impairment lasting several days. Support from family and antipyretic treatment (e.g., paracetamol) is recommended.

4. Very High Microfilaraemia (> 30,000 mf/ml):

In cases of very high microfilariae load, DEC should not be used due to risks of severe encephalopathy. Instead, microfilariae extraction may be considered, especially if an adult worm migrates to the conjunctiva.

Extraction of adult worms from the skin is not typically beneficial as they tend to die under the skin after DEC treatment.

Special Considerations:

If Loiasis is well-tolerated, treatment may not be necessary as the disease is typically benign. However, in symptomatic cases or when co-infected with onchocerciasis, ivermectin may be administered under strict medical supervision.

Albendazole can be used before administering DEC to reduce microfilaraemia, especially if DEC is contraindicated due to the risk of encephalopathy in patients with very high levels of microfilaraemia.

Contraindications for DEC:

High microfilaraemia (> 2,000 mf/ml): This increases the risk of encephalopathy, particularly with DEC treatment.

Co-infection with O. volvulus: The risk of severe eye lesions makes DEC unsuitable for these patients.

Pregnancy, infants, or patients in poor general condition: DEC is contraindicated in these groups.

Post-Treatment Complications:

Ivermectin side effects: Severe reactions such as encephalopathy may occur, typically within 2–3 days of administration, and are usually preceded by conjunctival hemorrhages. Symptoms are reversible with appropriate care and symptomatic treatment.

Monitoring is essential to manage any potential adverse

reactions, including encephalopathy, which requires supportive care and avoidance of steroids.

Footnotes

(a) Differential Diagnosis: Consider cutaneous larva .

(b) Pain Management: Some patients may experience severe pain, requiring assistance with daily activities. Regular monitoring is necessary to prevent complications like pressure sores.

(c) Ivermectin Encephalopathy: A severe reaction may occur between days 2-3 post-treatment. Symptoms are reversible with proper management. Avoid steroid use due to potential adverse effects.

Lymphatic Filariasis (LF)

Lymphatic filariasis (LF) is primarily distributed in tropical regions where mosquito vectors such as Anopheles, Culex, and Aedes thrive. The infection is predominantly caused by Wuchereria bancrofti (90% of cases) and, to a lesser extent, Brugia species (10%).

Clinical Features:

1. Acute Inflammatory Manifestations:
Adenolymphangitis: This condition involves painful, red, and swollen lymph nodes, often along the length of lymphatic channels. It may or may not be accompanied by systemic symptoms such as fever, nausea, and vomiting. The inflammation commonly affects the lower limbs, external genitalia, and breasts. In men, inflammation of the spermatic cord (funiculitis), epididymis, and testicle (epididymo-orchitis) is also common.
Resolution: Attacks typically resolve within a week but may recur regularly in chronic LF.
2. Chronic Manifestations:
Lymphoedema: This is swelling of the lower extremities, external genitalia, or breast caused by the blockage of lymphatic vessels by adult worms (microfilariae). Initially reversible, lymphoedema becomes progressively severe with skin thickening, hypertrophy of affected areas, and the formation of fibrous, verrucous lesions. The

final stage of lymphoedema is elephantiasis.

Genital Involvement: In men, chronic lymphoedema may cause hydrocele (accumulation of fluid around the testicles) and chronic epididymo-orchitis.

Chyluria: A condition where urine appears milky or contains a rice-water like appearance, caused by leakage of lymph into the urinary tract.

Infections: Co-infection with other filarial species like Brugia can present with less severe genital lesions and chyluria, typically with lymphoedema confined below the knee.

Laboratory Diagnosis:

Microfilariae Detection: Microfilariae can be detected in peripheral blood using a thick blood film. Specimens should be collected between 9 PM and 3 AM when microfilariae are most prevalent in the bloodstream.

Co-infections: In areas where Loa loa or volvulus are also present, screening for co-infections is recommended.

Treatment:

1. Antiparasitic Therapy:

Doxycycline: This antibiotic is effective for reducing the burden of adult worms and alleviating lymphoedema. A 4-week course of doxycycline (200 mg daily) is generally recommended. However, it is contraindicated in pregnant or breastfeeding women and children under 8 years old.

Diethylcarbamazine (DEC): A single dose of DEC (400 mg for adults and 3 mg/kg for children) can be used to treat LF. However, its effectiveness is variable and it does not significantly alleviate symptoms. Additionally, DEC is contraindicated in patients with Onchocerca or Loa loa co-infections, as well as in pregnant women.

2. Surgical Interventions:

Surgery may be necessary for severe cases of chronic lymphoedema, hydrocele, and chyluria, including procedures for diversion and reconstruction.

Hydrocele Management: Surgical options are also indicated for managing complications like hydrocele.

3. Acute Attack Management:

Rest and Elevation: Bed rest, limb elevation, and cooling (using wet cloths or cold baths) are recommended during acute episodes. Analgesics such as paracetamol can be used for pain, and antibacterial or antifungal creams may be applied if needed.
Hydration and Antipyretics: Ensuring adequate hydration and using antipyretics for fever is critical in managing acute symptoms.

4. Preventive Measures:

Hygiene and Footwear: Proper hygiene of affected limbs, wearing comfortable footwear, and immediate treatment of any secondary infections (bacterial or fungal) are important for preventing further complications.
Lymphoedema Management: Once lymphoedema becomes established, daily bandaging, limb elevation, and regular skin hygiene (washing with soap and water) are recommended. Exercises like foot flexion and ankle rotation can also help maintain lymphatic drainage.

Footnotes:

Differential Diagnosis: If standard test results are negative but the clinical presentation strongly suggests LF, additional diagnostic methods such as antigen detection using the ICT rapid test or ultrasound of the inguinal area (looking for the "filarial dance sign") should be considered.

Skin Care: Regular cleaning of the affected area (at least once a day) using soap and water is essential to prevent secondary infections and maintain skin integrity.

Chapter 7
Bacterial Diseases

This chapter covers a range of bacterial infections, including:

1. Bacterial Meningitis: Inflammation of the protective membranes of the brain and spinal cord caused by bacterial infection.

2. Tetanus: A serious infection caused by Clostridium tetani, leading to muscle stiffness and spasms.

3. Enteric Fevers (Typhoid and Paratyphoid): Systemic infections caused by Salmonella species, leading to fever, abdominal pain, and gastrointestinal symptoms.

4. Brucellosis: A zoonotic infection from Brucella species, causing fever, sweats, and muscle pain.
5. Plague: A deadly disease caused by Yersinia pestis, often spread by fleas, characterized by fever, lymph node swelling, and septicemia.
6. Leptospirosis: A bacterial infection spread by animals, presenting with flu-like symptoms and potentially severe complications.
7. Relapsing Fever (Borreliosis): Caused by Borrelia species, this fever recurs in episodes.
8. Louse-borne Relapsing Fever (LBRF): Transmitted by lice, this fever is characterized by recurring episodes of high fever.
9. Tick-borne Relapsing Fever (TBRF): A similar condition to LBRF but transmitted by ticks.
10. Eruptive Rickettsioses: A group of diseases caused by Rickettsia species, often associated with rashes and fever.

Bacterial Meningitis: Detailed Overview and Management
Introduction:
Bacterial meningitis is a severe infection of the meninges, the

protective membranes covering the brain and spinal cord, which can lead to serious complications such as neurological damage and hearing loss if not promptly treated. The condition is considered a medical emergency requiring rapid diagnosis and treatment.

Causes and Risk Factors:

The causative agents of bacterial meningitis vary based on age, geographical context, and underlying health conditions. Common pathogens include:

1. Neonates and Infants (0-2 months):
Group B Streptococcus
Escherichia coli
Klebsiella spp.

2. Children (3 months - 5 years):
Streptococcus pneumoniae
Haemophilus influenzae type b
Neisseria meningitidis

3. Children >5 years and Adults:
Streptococcus pneumoniae
Neisseria meningitidis

4. Special Populations:
Immunocompromised patients: Predominantly affected by Gram-negative bacilli and Mycobacterium tuberculosis.

Sickle cell anemia: Increased risk of infection with Salmonella spp. and Staphylococcus aureus.
Epidemic Context:
In regions like the Sahel, meningococcal meningitis epidemics (caused by Neisseria meningitidis serogroups A, C, or W135) often occur during the dry season. In these areas, children and adolescents are most vulnerable.
Clinical Presentation:
The symptoms of bacterial meningitis vary by age and clinical context, but the hallmark signs include:
In infants:
High fever, irritability, poor feeding, vomiting, altered consciousness, and bulging fontanelle.
In children (over 1 year) and adults:
Fever, headache, neck stiffness, photophobia, and altered mental status.
Classic signs like Brudzinski's sign and Kernig's sign may be present.
Purpuric rash may occur in meningococcal infections, with severe cases leading to seizures,

coma, and focal neurological deficits.
Diagnostic Workup:
The diagnosis of bacterial meningitis is confirmed via lumbar puncture (LP), where cerebrospinal fluid (CSF) analysis is essential. In endemic areas, it is crucial to test for concurrent diseases like malaria. The CSF findings in bacterial meningitis include:
Appearance: Cloudy or turbid CSF.
White Blood Cell (WBC) count: 100-20,000 cells/mm^3, predominantly neutrophils.
Protein levels: Typically elevated (>100 mg/dL).
Glucose levels: Decreased (often <40 mg/dL).
Gram stain: Positive for bacterial pathogens, although a negative result does not rule out infection.
Treatment in Non-Epidemic Context:
Immediate empirical antibiotic therapy is necessary to treat bacterial meningitis. Commonly used antibiotics include:
Neonates (0-28 days): Ampicillin plus cefotaxime or gentamicin.

Infants (1 month - 1 year): Ampicillin plus ceftriaxone or cefotaxime.
Children and adults: Ceftriaxone or cefotaxime plus vancomycin (to cover resistant organisms like Streptococcus pneumoniae).
Treatment duration varies based on the causative agent:
Neisseria and Haemophilus influenzae: 7 days.
Streptococcus pneumoniae: 10-14 days.
Gram-negative bacilli: 21 days.
In addition, dexamethasone may be administered to reduce the risk of hearing loss in infections caused by Haemophilus influenzae or Streptococcus pneumoniae, provided it is given before or with the first dose of antibiotics.
Treatment in Epidemic Context:
For meningococcal meningitis during an epidemic, a single dose of ceftriaxone (IM) is often recommended for those in close contact with infected individuals. If the case is confirmed but there is no improvement within 24 hours, the treatment is extended to a 5-day regimen of ceftriaxone.

Supportive Care:
Patients with meningitis require supportive care, including fluid management (oral or IV), nutritional support, and monitoring for complications such as seizures or coma. Preventative measures, including pressure ulcer care and eye/mouth hygiene, are also critical.

Conclusion:
Bacterial meningitis remains a critical medical condition requiring prompt intervention. Early diagnosis, appropriate antibiotic therapy, and supportive care are essential in reducing mortality and long-term complications such as hearing loss and neurological deficits. The treatment protocol varies depending on age, causative pathogens, and whether the case occurs in an epidemic setting.

Footnotes
(a) For intramuscular (IM) administration, the total dose may be divided into two injections, with half of the dose administered in each buttock if necessary.

References

1. van de Beek, D., Cabellos, C., Dzuppova, O., Esposito, S., Klein, M., Kloek, A.T., Leib, S.L., Mourvillier, B., Ostergaard, C., Pagliano, P., Pfister, H.W., Read, R.C., Sipahi, O.R., Brouwer, M.C. ESCMID guideline: diagnosis and treatment of acute bacterial meningitis, 2016. Clinical Microbiology and Infection. Available at: https://www.clinicalmicrobiologyandinfection.com/article/S1198-743X(16)00020-3/pdf
2. Kaplan, S.L. Bacterial meningitis in children: Dexamethasone and other measures to prevent neurologic complications. UpToDate, Accessed February 25, 2019.
3. World Health Organization. Managing meningitis epidemics in Africa: A quick reference guide for health authorities and health-care workers, 2015. Available at: https://apps.who.int/iris/bitstream/handle/10665/154595/WHO_HSE_GAR_ERI_2010.4_Rev1_eng.pdf?sequence=

Tetanus: Overview, Clinical Features, and Management

Introduction Tetanus is a potentially life-threatening infection caused by Clostridium tetani, a bacterium found in soil and animal feces. The infection occurs when the bacteria enter the body through wounds, releasing a potent toxin that impacts the central nervous system. Notably, tetanus is not contagious.

Tetanus is preventable through vaccination. Individuals who are not fully vaccinated or have not received adequate post-exposure prophylaxis are at risk. The condition is commonly associated with injuries such as puncture wounds, burns, bites, and certain surgical procedures performed under non-sterile conditions.

Clinical Features The most common and severe form of tetanus is generalized tetanus. Symptoms typically begin with muscular rigidity, starting in the jaw muscles (trismus), making it difficult for the patient to speak or eat. The rigidity then spreads to the neck, face, trunk, and limbs, with the patient eventually experiencing painful muscle spasms. Despite these symptoms, the patient's level of consciousness generally remains intact.

In neonates, the first signs include irritability and difficulty sucking, followed by muscle rigidity and spasms. If a neonate presents with these symptoms within 3 to 28 days after birth, neonatal tetanus should be suspected.

Tetanus treatment typically requires hospitalization, often for 3 to 4 weeks. Early and appropriate management can significantly reduce mortality rates, even in hospitals with limited resources. The management approach is multifaceted, including general measures, neutralization of the toxin, inhibition of toxin production, and controlling muscle spasms.

1. General Measures:

Intensive nursing care is essential, with the patient placed in a dark, quiet room.

Sedation and minimal handling are necessary to reduce stimulus-induced spasms.

IV access should be established for hydration and medication administration.
Nutritional support is crucial, with neonates receiving expressed breast milk every 3 hours.

2. Neutralization of Toxin:

Human tetanus immunoglobulin (500 IU) should be administered IM in two separate sites to neutralize the toxin.

3. Inhibition of Toxin Production:

Metronidazole (IV infusion) is used to inhibit the bacteria's toxin production. The dosage depends on the age and weight of the patient. For neonates, metronidazole is administered at a dose of 15 mg/kg on Day 1, followed by 7.5 mg/kg every 12 hours. For children over 1 month, the dose is 10 mg/kg every 8 hours.

4. Control of Muscle Rigidity and Spasms:

Diazepam is the primary drug used to control spasms. It is administered either intravenously or orally, depending on the patient's age and condition. Close monitoring of respiratory rate and oxygen saturation is critical to avoid respiratory depression, especially in children and elderly patients.

5. Pain Management:

Morphine may be used to manage severe pain. However, caution is required when administering morphine with diazepam due to the increased risk of respiratory depression.

6. Wound Care:

Proper wound care is essential for tetanus management. This includes cleaning, debridement, and disinfection of the entry wound. In cases of neonatal tetanus, infections at the umbilical stump require treatment for bacterial omphalitis and sepsis with antibiotics such as cloxacillin or gentamicin.

Vaccination and Prevention

Tetanus prevention is primarily through vaccination. The vaccine is highly effective when administered as part of a series of three or more doses. Post-exposure prophylaxis is also essential for individuals with incomplete vaccination or those who are at risk due to a recent injury.

For neonates with tetanus, it is vital to vaccinate the mother as well. When tetanus occurs in an individual, tetanus vaccination should be administered once the patient has recovered.

Post-exposure Prophylaxis: For individuals with incomplete tetanus vaccination, tetanus immunoglobulin and vaccination should be administered after exposure. This will prevent the development of symptoms or reduce their severity.

Conclusion Tetanus remains a critical infection that can be effectively prevented through vaccination. Immediate and correct management of the infection, including toxin neutralization, muscle spasm control, and supportive care, is vital to improving outcomes. Preventive measures, including vaccination and proper wound care, are key to reducing the incidence of tetanus worldwide.

Footnotes

(a) Clindamycin administered intravenously for seven days can be considered as an alternative treatment option (refer to "Periorbital and Orbital

Cellulitis," Chapter 5, for dosing details).
(b) When giving oral diazepam to infants, ensure precise dosing. For instance, to administer 0.5 mg of diazepam, divide a scored 2 mg tablet in half, then cut one half into two quarters. Crush one quarter and dissolve it in expressed breast milk or infant formula.
(c) Signs of withdrawal may include excessive irritability, tremors, heightened muscle tone, frequent yawning, poor feeding, watery stools, and sweating.
(d) The tetanus-containing vaccine, such as Td, DTP, DTP + HepB, or DTP + HepB + Hib, should be administered based on availability and the patient's needs.

Enteric Fevers: Typhoid and Paratyphoid
Last Updated: March 2024
Enteric fevers, which include typhoid fever caused by Salmonella enterica serotype Typhi (S. Typhi) and paratyphoid fever due to Salmonella enterica serotypes Paratyphi A, B, or C (S. Paratyphi), are infectious diseases typically acquired by

consuming water or food contaminated with the feces of symptomatic or asymptomatic carriers. Direct contact with contaminated hands can also facilitate transmission.

These fevers are endemic in regions such as South, Central, and Southeast Asia, Sub-Saharan Africa, Oceania, and, to a lesser extent, Latin America. Timely and appropriate treatment is crucial, as it significantly reduces the risk of complications and mortality.

Clinical Features

The symptoms of typhoid and paratyphoid fevers are similar, with the disease typically presenting in a gradual and insidious manner. The clinical course can range from mild to severe. The primary feature is prolonged fever, which increases over the first week, stabilizes during the second week, and typically begins to decrease in the third to fourth week.

Non-specific symptoms often accompany the fever, including gastrointestinal disturbances (such as abdominal pain, constipation, diarrhea, or vomiting), headache, malaise, chills, fatigue, and a nonproductive cough. Hepatosplenomegaly is also common. Additionally, some patients may develop a characteristic erythematous maculopapular rash on the trunk, extreme fatigue, and relative bradycardia (a dissociation between heart rate and temperature).

Serious complications can affect up to 27% of hospitalized patients, usually manifesting during the second or third week of illness. These complications include altered mental status, intestinal hemorrhage or perforation, peritonitis, shock, and nephritis. Pregnant women may experience additional risks, such as miscarriage, preterm delivery, or intrauterine death.

Relapses can occur 2-3 weeks after apparent recovery, which are typically not related to antibiotic resistance but still require re-treatment.

Differential Diagnosis

Because enteric fevers often resemble other infectious diseases common in endemic areas, clinical diagnosis can be challenging. Key differential diagnoses include malaria, brucellosis, leptospirosis, typhus, rickettsiosis, sepsis, and dengue.

Laboratory Diagnosis

The gold standard for diagnosing enteric fevers is culturing S. Typhi or S. Paratyphi from blood or stool specimens, alongside performing a drug susceptibility test. In malaria-endemic regions, a rapid malaria test is essential, with appropriate treatment initiated as needed (refer to Chapter 6 on Malaria). However, serological tests, such as the Widal agglutination test, are not recommended due to their low sensitivity and specificity.

Treatment

General Approach

Hydration and fever management are essential in all cases. Antibiotics are the cornerstone of treatment, with fever typically resolving within 4 to 5 days after the initiation of effective antibiotic therapy. The choice of antibiotic should be based on the local resistance patterns and national guidelines. Resistance to first-line antibiotics like chloramphenicol, ampicillin, and co-trimoxazole (multidrug-resistant or MDR strains) is widespread in many regions, and newer antibiotics may be required.

First-line antibiotics include:

Azithromycin (7-day oral course) is effective for both MDR and extensively drug-resistant (XDR) strains, as well as in pregnant women.

Pediatric dose: 10-20 mg/kg (max 1g) once daily.

Adult dose: 500 mg to 1g once daily, or 1g on Day 1 followed by 500 mg once daily.

Cefixime (10-14 day oral course), except in cases of resistance to third-generation cephalosporins or XDR strains.

Pediatric dose: 10 mg/kg (max 200 mg) twice daily.

Adult dose: 200 mg twice daily.

Alternative antibiotics (if local resistance data support their efficacy):

Amoxicillin (14-day oral course).

Pediatric dose: 30 mg/kg (max 1g) 3 times daily.

Adult dose: 1g 3 times daily.

Co-trimoxazole (14-day oral course).

Pediatric dose: 20 mg SMX + 4 mg TMP/kg (max 800 mg SMX + 160 mg TMP) twice daily.
Adult dose: 800 mg SMX + 160 mg TMP twice daily.

Severe Cases

In severe cases, such as those with a toxic appearance, decreased consciousness, or complications like intestinal hemorrhage, initial treatment should be parenteral. Ceftriaxone is commonly used:

Pediatric dose: 50 to 100 mg/kg (max 4g) once daily.
Adult dose: 2g once or twice daily.

If ceftriaxone resistance or XDR strains are suspected, meropenem should be administered intravenously, followed by a switch to oral azithromycin for a full 7-day course.

In cases of shock, severe mental status changes, or intestinal perforation, dexamethasone may be administered: a loading dose of 1 mg/kg, followed by 0.25 mg/kg every 6 hours for 48 hours (a total of 8 doses). If perforation or peritonitis is suspected, urgent surgical consultation and metronidazole for anaerobic coverage may be required.

Prevention and Hygiene

Prevention of enteric fevers revolves around maintaining good hygiene practices, such as regular handwashing, consuming treated water (chlorinated, boiled, or bottled), and ensuring food is adequately washed and cooked. In healthcare settings, particularly for patients with watery diarrhea, excreta should be disinfected with a chlorinated solution.

Vaccination with the typhoid conjugate vaccine is recommended in endemic areas, particularly during outbreaks. However, this vaccine does not provide protection against paratyphoid fever.

Footnotes

(a) Ceftriaxone for IM injection should never be administered intravenously if reconstituted with lidocaine. For intravenous administration, always use water for injection.

(b) Do not combine metronidazole with meropenem as meropenem already covers anaerobic bacteria.

(c) For further details on typhoid vaccines, see the WHO position paper: WHO Typhoid Vaccines Paper.

References

1. Cruz Espinoza LM, McCreedy E, Holm M, et al. Occurrence of typhoid fever complications and their relation to duration of illness preceding hospitalization: a systematic literature review and meta-analysis. Clin Infect Dis. 2019;69(Suppl 6):S435-48. PMC6821330 [Accessed 28 June 2022].

2. Browne AJ, Hamadani BHK, Kumaran EAP, Rao P, et al. Drug-resistant enteric fever worldwide, 1990 to 2018: a systematic review and meta-analysis. BMC Medicine. 2020;18:1+22. DOI: 10.1186/s12916-019-1443-1 [Accessed 23 February 2022].

3. Klemm EJ, Shakoor S, Page AJ, Qamar FN, et al. Emergence of an Extensively Drug-Resistant Salmonella enterica Serovar Typhi Clone Harboring a Promiscuous Plasmid Encoding Resistance to Fluoroquinolones and Third-Generation Cephalosporins. mBio. 2018 Jan-

Feb; 9(1): e00105-18. PMC5821095 [Accessed 26 June 2022].

Brucellosis: A Comprehensive Overview

Overview: Brucellosis is a zoonotic disease primarily affecting livestock, caused by bacteria of the Brucella genus, such as B. (sheep and goats), B. abortus (cattle), and B. (pigs). The disease is prevalent globally, particularly in rural regions. Brucellosis can cause recurrent infections and may evolve into chronic forms despite initial treatment. The transmission to humans occurs primarily through consumption of unpasteurized milk products, direct contact with infected animals, or their carcasses.

Clinical Presentation:

Acute Brucellosis: Initial infection often presents with a range of non-specific symptoms, making diagnosis challenging. Patients commonly experience fluctuating fever (39-40°C), chills, night sweats, fatigue, malaise, muscle and joint pain, weight loss, and headaches. In some cases, there may be associated adenopathy, gastrointestinal issues, cough, and hepatosplenomegaly.

Localized Infections: In rare cases, brucellosis may progress to more localized infections, manifesting months or even years after the primary infection. The common sites affected include the osteoarticular system (sacroiliac joint, lower limb joints, and spine), genitourinary system (orchitis, epididymitis), and neurological system (meningitis, encephalitis).

Diagnostic Approaches:

Blood Culture: The gold standard for diagnosis, though Brucella cultures are slow-growing (7-21 days), making early detection challenging.

Serological Tests: Tests such as the Rose Bengal test, Wright agglutination test, and ELISA can aid in presumptive diagnosis.

Neurological Involvement: Lumbar puncture may show elevated white blood cells and protein in cerebrospinal fluid with decreased glucose levels, suggesting possible meningitis.

Radiographic Imaging: Used to assess the extent of organ

involvement, particularly in the case of osteoarticular brucellosis.

Treatment Strategies: The treatment regimen for brucellosis typically involves a combination of antibiotics for an extended period, ranging from 6 weeks to 4 months depending on the infection's localization.

Standard Antibiotics:

Co-trimoxazole: For pediatric patients under 8 years, the dosage is 20 mg SMX + 4 mg TMP/kg, administered twice daily.

Doxycycline: Given for 6 weeks, starting at a dose of 2-2.2 mg/kg for children over 8 years or adults.

Rifampicin: Administered for 6 weeks at a dose of 600 to 900 mg daily for adults.

Gentamicin or Streptomycin: These are used as adjunctive therapies, typically for the first 2 weeks of treatment.

Prevention Measures: Preventive strategies include:

Proper handling of livestock and their products, including avoiding consumption of unpasteurized milk.

Washing hands and clothes after animal contact.

Ensuring that animal carcasses are properly disposed of, and avoiding direct contact with infected animals.

Plague: An In-Depth Examination

Overview: Plague is a serious zoonotic disease caused by the bacterium Yersinia pestis, which primarily infects wild rodents. The disease can be transmitted to humans via flea bites or direct contact with infected animal tissues. The pneumonic form can also spread person-to-person through respiratory droplets. Natural foci of plague include Africa, Asia, North and South America, and parts of Europe.

Clinical Manifestations:

Bubonic Plague: The most common form, usually acquired through flea bites. Symptoms include fever, chills, malaise, and painful swollen lymph nodes (buboes), most commonly in the inguinal region. If untreated, the bacteria can spread, leading to more severe forms of plague.

Pneumonic Plague: Characterized by severe

respiratory symptoms including cough, chest pain, and difficulty breathing. It can progress rapidly to respiratory failure and shock if not treated promptly.

Septicemic Plague: A life-threatening form that may present with systemic symptoms such as gastrointestinal distress (vomiting, diarrhea) and can rapidly progress to disseminated intravascular coagulation (DIC), shock, and death.

Plague Meningitis: A rare but severe complication where the infection spreads to the central nervous system, causing symptoms like headache, fever, and stiff neck.

Differential Diagnosis: Key conditions to differentiate from plague include bacterial lymphadenitis, tularemia, malaria (in endemic areas), and other causes of acute pneumonia and septicemia.

Diagnostic Techniques:

Specimen Collection: Depending on the form of plague, samples from lymph nodes (bubonic), sputum (mnemonic), blood (septicemic), or cerebrospinal

fluid (plague meningitis) are essential for diagnosis.
Laboratory Tests:
Rapid diagnostic tests for detecting the F1 antigen of Y. pestis.
PCR assays for genetic identification.
Cultures to isolate Y. pestis, followed by drug susceptibility testing.
Treatment Protocols: Empiric antibiotic therapy should be initiated immediately if plague is suspected, even before laboratory confirmation.
First-line Treatment:
Doxycycline: Preferred for its efficacy against Y. pestis.
Gentamicin: Often used for more severe forms of plague.
Ciprofloxacin: An alternative for non-severe cases.
In cases of pneumonic plague, more aggressive combination therapy (e.g., doxycycline + gentamicin) may be required.
For plague meningitis, treatment should include a combination of chloramphenicol and ciprofloxacin or gentamicin.
Prevention Measures:

Vector Control: Flea eradication is critical in preventing human-to-human transmission. Rodent population control is also essential in plague-endemic regions.
Post-Exposure Prophylaxis: If exposure occurs, immediate prophylactic antibiotics (e.g., doxycycline or ciprofloxacin) should be administered to prevent disease onset.
Vaccination: Although not widely used, vaccination is recommended for laboratory workers and those at high risk of exposure.
Conclusion: Both brucellosis and plague are serious infectious diseases with significant public health implications. Timely diagnosis and appropriate treatment are crucial in preventing complications and death. Proactive prevention strategies, including proper hygiene, vector control, and public health measures, are essential for reducing transmission risk, especially in endemic regions.
Footnotes

(a) When transporting specimens in 0.9% sodium chloride, it is essential to maintain a cold chain. If a cold chain is not possible, the temperature must remain below 30°C. Additionally, triple packaging and proper labeling with UN3373 are required.

References

1. Nelson CA, Meaney-Delman D, Fleck-Derderian S, Cooley KM, et al. Antimicrobial treatment and prophylaxis of plague: recommendations for naturally acquired infection and bioterrorism response. MMWR Recomm Rep. 2021;70(No. RR-3):1-27.

Plague Overview

Plague is a zoonotic disease caused by Yersinia pestis, a Gram-negative bacterium that primarily affects rodents but can also infect other mammals. The disease can be transmitted to humans through various means, including direct contact with infected animals or their respiratory droplets, flea bites, and exposure to respiratory droplets from individuals suffering from pneumonic plague.

Plague naturally occurs in certain regions, including parts of Africa, Asia, North and South America, and Europe. The most common form of the disease is bubonic plague, which typically results from the bite of an infected flea. Without prompt medical intervention, the infection may spread through the bloodstream, causing severe complications such as pneumonic plague, which carries a high mortality rate if untreated.

Forms of Plague

1. Bubonic Plague: This is the most common form, marked by fever, chills, malaise, and headache. A painful swelling of the lymph nodes, usually in the groin, is characteristic. If untreated, the bacteria can spread hematogenously, leading to more severe forms like septicemic or pneumonic plague.

2. Pneumonic Plague: This form affects the lungs, leading to respiratory distress, chest pain, cough, and the production of purulent or blood-stained sputum. Without rapid treatment,

it can progress quickly to respiratory failure and septic shock, resulting in high mortality.

3. Septicaemic Plague: This severe form of plague can cause disseminated intravascular coagulation (DIC), shock, and organ failure. Symptoms may include gastrointestinal issues like abdominal pain, vomiting, and diarrhea, with no localized symptoms at the onset.

4. Plague Meningitis: Although rare, this is a severe and often fatal form of plague involving inflammation of the membranes surrounding the brain and spinal cord.

Differential Diagnosis

Plague should be differentiated from other diseases that cause lymphadenitis, acute pneumonia, sepsis, or meningitis. Some of these include bacterial skin infections, tularemia, and other causes of bacterial meningitis and sepsis.

Laboratory Diagnosis

Diagnostic tests are essential for confirming plague. Pre-treatment specimens should be collected, including:

Bubonic plague: Lymph node aspirate
Pneumonic plague: Sputum
Septicaemic plague: Blood
Plague meningitis: Cerebrospinal fluid
Laboratory confirmation can be achieved using:
Rapid diagnostic tests detecting the F1 capsular antigen of Y. pestis
PCR assays
Culturing Y. pestis followed by drug susceptibility testing
In endemic regions, a rapid malaria test should be performed, and treatment for malaria should be administered if necessary.
Management
Empiric Treatment: Upon suspicion of plague, empiric antibiotics should be administered immediately, ideally within 24 hours of symptom onset, to reduce mortality. A 10 to 14-day course of antibiotics is typically recommended. A combination of two antibiotics from different classes should be used in severe cases, including plague meningitis and in pregnant women.

The recommended treatments include:
Bubonic plague: Doxycycline, gentamicin, or ciprofloxacin
Pneumonic plague: Gentamicin, ciprofloxacin, or doxycycline, depending on the severity
Septicaemic plague: Same as pneumonic plague, with intensive care support as needed
Plague meningitis: Chloramphenicol IV plus ciprofloxacin or gentamicin
Pregnant Women: Antibiotics must be chosen carefully to avoid harm to the fetus. Streptomycin is contraindicated in pregnancy, but gentamicin and doxycycline are considered safer alternatives.
Post-exposure Prophylaxis
People who have had close contact with a pneumonic plague patient or contaminated bodily fluids should receive post-exposure prophylaxis. Treatment options include:
Doxycycline or ciprofloxacin for 7 days, depending on age and health status.
Infection Control
In healthcare settings, patients with pneumonic plague should be isolated, ideally in a single

room, and healthcare workers should use droplet precautions for 48 hours after the initiation of antibiotic therapy. For aerosol-generating procedures, airborne precautions should be employed.

Flea and Rodent Control: Prevention efforts focus on controlling flea vectors and rodent reservoirs. This includes ensuring sanitation and eliminating flea-infested bedding or clothing.

Vaccination: While there is a vaccine for individuals working with Y. pestis in laboratories, it is not recommended for use in epidemic settings.

References

1. Nelson CA, Meaney-Delman D, Fleck-Derderian S, Cooley KM, et al. Antimicrobial treatment and prophylaxis of plague: recommendations for naturally acquired infection and bioterrorism response. MMWR Recomm Rep. 2021;70(No. RR-3):1-27.

Leptospirosis: Overview and Management

Leptospirosis is a zoonotic infection caused by spirochete bacteria of the Leptospira genus.

It primarily affects animals, particularly rodents like rats, as well as dogs, cattle, and other wildlife. Humans typically acquire the infection through direct contact with the urine or bodily fluids of infected animals, either through broken skin or mucous membranes (such as the eyes or mouth). This disease is found worldwide, with higher incidence in tropical and subtropical regions, and is often associated with outbreaks following heavy rainfall or flooding.

Clinical Presentation

Leptospirosis manifests in two forms: mild and severe.

1. Mild Form: Most cases (around 90%) are asymptomatic or cause mild symptoms. These include fever, headache, muscle aches, and conjunctival suffusion (redness of the eyes without discharge). The symptoms may resolve on their own without complications.

2. Severe (Ictero-haemorrhagic) Form: In 5-15% of cases, the infection can progress to a more severe form characterized by organ dysfunction, including

renal failure (oliguria or polyuria), liver damage (jaundice), and widespread hemorrhages (such as purpura, epistaxis, or hemoptysis). Cardiac and pulmonary involvement, such as myocarditis and chest pain, can also occur. Without timely treatment, the severe form carries a high risk of mortality.

The progression of leptospirosis is divided into two phases:

Acute Phase (Septicaemic): This phase is marked by a sudden onset of high fever, chills, muscle pain (especially in the calves and lower back), headache, and photophobia. The hallmark of this phase is conjunctival suffusion, a reddening of the eyes without discharge. Other symptoms may include gastrointestinal distress (nausea, vomiting, anorexia), non-productive cough, and hepatomegaly.

Immune Phase: After 5-7 days, symptoms often improve but can re-emerge in a milder form. However, signs of meningitis, thought to be immune-mediated, are common during this phase.

Diagnosis

The diagnosis of leptospirosis is challenging due to the wide range of clinical manifestations that overlap with other infectious diseases. Key diagnostic indicators include:

A sudden onset of fever, chills, headache, muscle pain, and jaundice

A history of exposure to contaminated environments, such as swimming or working in floodwaters, rice fields, or farms

Risk factors such as close contact with infected animals (e.g., veterinarians, farmers, and slaughterhouse workers)

Differential diagnoses include viral hemorrhagic fevers (e.g., dengue, Zika), malaria, brucellosis, typhoid fever, and rickettsioses. Laboratory tests for leptospirosis may include:

Serology: Detection of IgM antibodies through ELISA or microscopic agglutination test (MAT) during the acute and immune phases.

PCR: For detection of Leptospira DNA, especially during the early stages of illness.

Urine analysis: Proteinuria, leukocyturia, and microscopic hematuria can be seen during the acute phase.

Treatment

Leptospirosis treatment is primarily antibiotic-based and should begin as soon as the disease is suspected, even before definitive diagnosis.

Mild cases (outpatients): Symptomatic treatment is often sufficient. Antibiotic regimens for mild cases include doxycycline or penicillin. The usual dosage for children and adults depends on body weight and clinical condition, with special dosing considerations for pregnant women.

Severe cases (inpatients): Hospitalization is necessary for severe cases, and treatment focuses on stabilizing the patient, managing organ dysfunction, and addressing complications such as shock and renal failure. Antibiotics such as ceftriaxone or doxycycline are given intravenously. Supportive care is essential, including fluid management for oliguria, and treatment of complications like bleeding or liver dysfunction.

In rare cases, antibiotics may provoke a Jarisch-Herxheimer reaction (a temporary worsening of symptoms, including fever, chills, and hypotension) that requires careful monitoring.

Prevention

Preventive measures include:

Avoiding contact with freshwater in endemic areas, particularly during floods.

Wearing protective clothing (e.g., rubber boots and gloves) when in environments where animal urine contamination is likely.

Disinfecting objects and laundry contaminated by urine from infected animals or humans.

Vaccination is available for animals but not routinely recommended for humans, except for those at high risk (e.g., workers in high-risk environments).

Conclusion

Leptospirosis is a potentially severe infectious disease with a wide range of clinical presentations. Early recognition, prompt treatment with

antibiotics, and supportive care are key to improving patient outcomes. Preventive measures, particularly avoiding contact with contaminated water sources, are critical in reducing the risk of infection.
Footnote
(a) For intravenous administration of ceftriaxone, dilute with water for injection only.

Relapsing Fever (Borreliosis)
Overview
Relapsing fever (FR) is a bacterial infection caused by Borrelia spirochetes, transmitted to humans via arthropod vectors. It includes two distinct forms:
1. Louse-borne Relapsing Fever (LBRF):
Etiology and Epidemiology: Caused by Borrelia , LBRF occurs primarily in overcrowded, unsanitary conditions such as refugee camps and prisons. Endemic regions include Sudan and the Horn of Africa, especially Ethiopia. LBRF is frequently associated with louse-borne typhus.
Clinical Manifestations: Symptoms begin with high fever,

headache, severe muscle and joint pain, chills, and gastrointestinal issues. The fever is followed by a "crisis" phase, marked by a sudden rise in body temperature and heart rate, followed by a drastic drop. The cycle repeats, with each episode becoming milder.

Diagnosis: Diagnosis is confirmed by detecting Borrelia spirochetes in blood smears during febrile episodes, as spirochetes are absent during febrile periods.

Treatment: Antibiotics, such as doxycycline (200 mg for adults), erythromycin, or azithromycin, are used for treatment. Adequate management of fever and pain, along with dehydration prevention, is crucial. Body lice control is essential to prevent outbreaks.

Complications: Untreated cases can result in complications like myocarditis, cerebral hemorrhage, and, during pregnancy, fetal death.

2. Tick-borne Relapsing Fever (TBRF):

Etiology and Epidemiology: TBRF is caused by various

Borrelia species and is endemic in temperate and tropical regions, particularly in rural Africa. It is a significant cause of illness, especially among children and pregnant women. The mortality rate for untreated TBRF ranges from 2% to 15%.
Clinical Manifestations: Symptoms include recurring fevers, similar to LBRF, with an increased incidence of central nervous system involvement, particularly lymphocytic meningitis. The disease often mimics other tropical diseases, such as malaria or typhoid fever.
Diagnosis: Blood tests identifying Borrelia spirochetes during febrile episodes confirm the diagnosis. Malaria tests are recommended in endemic areas to rule out co-infection.
Treatment: First-line treatment includes doxycycline (100 mg twice daily for adults) or azithromycin if doxycycline is contraindicated. In cases of CNS involvement or pregnancy, ceftriaxone is recommended.
Complications: Like LBRF, TBRF can lead to severe

neurological outcomes, including meningitis.

Both forms of relapsing fever are characterized by cyclic febrile episodes and necessitate timely antibiotic therapy to prevent complications. Close monitoring for Jarisch-Herxheimer reactions, particularly after antibiotic administration, is important in managing these infections.

Footnotes

(a) For IV administration of ceftriaxone, dilute only with water for injection.

Chapter 8
Viral Diseases

This chapter explores significant viral diseases, including their epidemiology, clinical features, and management strategies. Topics covered include:

1. Measles – A highly contagious viral infection characterized by fever, rash, and respiratory symptoms.

2. Poliomyelitis – A debilitating viral disease affecting the nervous system, potentially causing paralysis.

3. Rabies – A fatal viral encephalitis transmitted through animal bites.

4. Viral Hepatitis – Infections caused by various hepatitis viruses, leading to liver inflammation and complications.
5. Dengue – A mosquito-borne viral illness presenting with fever, rash, and potential hemorrhagic manifestations.
6. Viral Haemorrhagic Fevers – Severe, often fatal illnesses, such as Ebola and Marburg, marked by vascular damage and bleeding.
7. HIV Infection and AIDS – A progressive viral disease compromising the immune system, increasing susceptibility to opportunistic infections and malignancies.

Measles: A Detailed Analysis

Overview

Measles is a highly contagious viral disease transmitted primarily through respiratory droplets from infected individuals. Predominantly affecting children under five years of age, measles is preventable through vaccination programs. Effective management and prevention rely on early recognition, vaccination strategies, and comprehensive case management during outbreaks.

Clinical Presentation

Measles manifests through distinct clinical stages:

1. Incubation Period

Duration: Approximately 10 days.

Patients remain asymptomatic during this phase.

2. Prodromal Phase (2–4 Days)

Characterized by fever, cough, nasal discharge, and conjunctivitis.

Koplik's spots, bluish-white lesions on an erythematous base, may appear on the inner cheeks, serving as a hallmark of measles.

3. Eruptive Phase (4–6 Days)

Erythematous maculopapular rash appears, typically starting on the forehead and spreading downward.

Rash progression correlates with subsidence of initial symptoms.

The eruption resolves in the order it appeared, followed by skin desquamation lasting 1–2 weeks.

4. Complications

Pneumonia and dehydration are leading causes of mortality.

Other complications include otitis media, laryngotracheobronchitis, keratitis, xerophthalmia, diarrhea, febrile seizures, and encephalitis.

Post-measles malnutrition is a significant concern in resource-limited settings.

Diagnosis

A clinical diagnosis is based on fever, maculopapular rash, and at least one associated symptom such as cough, conjunctivitis, or nasal discharge. Laboratory confirmation is not routinely required but may be used for epidemiological studies.

Case Management

Management of measles requires a dual approach encompassing supportive care and treatment of complications:

1. Supportive Treatment

Fever Management: Use of paracetamol.

Hydration: Oral rehydration solutions or intravenous fluids for dehydration.

Nutritional Support: Frequent meals and supplementation with vitamin A to prevent ocular complications.

Isolation: Infected individuals should remain isolated to limit transmission.

2. Treatment of Complications

Severe Pneumonia: Administration of ceftriaxone with oxygen therapy if hypoxia is present.

Otitis Media: Amoxicillin for 5 days.

Ocular Complications: Tetracycline eye ointment and vitamin A supplementation.

Neurological Issues: Management of febrile seizures with antipyretics and supportive care.

Prevention

Vaccination remains the cornerstone of measles prevention:

Routine Immunization: The World Health Organization (WHO) recommends two doses, with the first dose at 9–12 months and the second dose at 15–18 months.

High-Risk Settings: Infants as young as six months can receive an additional dose during outbreaks or in high-risk areas, followed by the standard schedule.

Catch-Up Vaccination: Individuals under 15 years who missed routine doses should be vaccinated during healthcare visits.

Poliomyelitis: Comprehensive Review

Overview

Poliomyelitis, caused by poliovirus serotypes 1, 2, or 3, is an acute viral infection transmitted via the fecal-oral route. Humans are the sole reservoir, making eradication achievable through mass immunization programs. While most cases are asymptomatic, the paralytic form can lead to life-threatening complications.

Clinical Features

1. Asymptomatic or Mild Cases:
Up to 90% of infections present with mild, nonspecific symptoms such as fever, muscle pain, and gastrointestinal disturbances.

2. Paralytic Form (Rare, <1% Cases):
Rapid onset of asymmetrical acute flaccid paralysis, predominantly in the lower limbs.

Paralysis may ascend, affecting respiratory and swallowing muscles.

Muscle weakness is accompanied by reduced reflexes, with sensation typically preserved.

Diagnosis

Stool samples collected within 14 days of symptom onset are analyzed for poliovirus.

Active surveillance is essential for detecting acute flaccid paralysis (AFP), as each AFP case corresponds to numerous subclinical infections.

Treatment

1. Supportive Care:

Bed rest and prevention of bedsores.

Mechanical ventilation for respiratory muscle paralysis.

Physiotherapy to prevent muscle atrophy and contractures.

2. Outbreak Response:

Immediate mass vaccination within affected areas, targeting all children under five years.

Two additional rounds of mass vaccination are conducted to ensure coverage and interruption of virus transmission.

Door-to-door campaigns may be necessary to reach missed populations.

Prevention

Polio vaccination protocols vary by region, but the WHO recommends:

Primary Vaccination Schedule:

Birth: bivalent oral polio vaccine (bOPV).

6, 10, and 14 weeks: bOPV with inactivated polio vaccine (IPV) at 14 weeks.

Catch-Up Immunization:

Administer IPV alongside bOPV for children who initiate vaccination late.

Ensure complete immunization through mass campaigns in endemic regions.

Transition to IPV:

Long-term plans aim to replace bOPV with IPV to reduce vaccine-derived polio risks.

References

1. World Health Organization. Poliomyelitis (Polio). Available at: https://www.who.int/health-topics/poliomyelitis#tab=tab_1. Accessed June 8, 2021.

2. Centers for Disease Control and Prevention. Poliomyelitis: The Pink Book - Epidemiology

and Prevention of Vaccine-Preventable Diseases. 2020. Available at: https://www.cdc.gov/vaccines/pubs/pinkbook/polio.html. Accessed June 8, 2021.
3. Global Polio Eradication Initiative. Standard Operating Procedures for Responding to Poliovirus Events and Outbreaks, Version 3.1. World Health Organization. 2020. Available at: https://www.who.int/publications/i/item/9789240002999. Accessed June 8, 2021.

Rabies: Comprehensive Overview and Management

Introduction

Rabies is a zoonotic viral infection affecting both wild and domestic mammals, with humans becoming infected primarily through the saliva of infected animals. Transmission occurs via bites, scratches, or contact with broken skin and mucous membranes. This disease is prevalent in endemic regions, such as Africa and Asia, where dogs are responsible for approximately 99% of human cases. Children under 15 years account for nearly 40% of all cases in these areas.

Disease Progression

Rabies is entirely preventable through timely administration of post-exposure prophylaxis (PEP) before symptom onset. However, once clinical symptoms emerge, the disease is invariably fatal, and treatment becomes palliative.

Clinical Presentation

The diagnosis of rabies can be challenging due to the potential lack of a clear history of exposure, as minor scratches or licks may be overlooked, and wounds might have healed by the time of evaluation. The disease progresses through the following stages:

1. Incubation Period: Typically ranges from 20 to 90 days but can vary based on the severity and location of exposure. Severe exposures, such as bites on the face or hands, may result in shorter incubation periods, whereas 20% of patients develop symptoms after 90 days and a small fraction more than a year later.

2. Prodromal Phase: Initial symptoms include localized

itching, paresthesia, or neuropathic pain around the exposure site, often accompanied by nonspecific systemic symptoms like fever and malaise.

3. Neurological Phase:

Encephalitic (Furious) Rabies: Characterized by agitation, hydrophobia (panic and throat spasms triggered by water stimuli), aerophobia, and potential seizures. Periods of lucidity may alternate with episodes of psychomotor excitement. Paralysis and coma ensue in advanced stages.

Paralytic Rabies: A rarer form (20% of cases) resembling Guillain-Barré syndrome with progressive ascending paralysis, eventually leading to coma.

Post-Exposure Prophylaxis (PEP)

WHO Exposure Categories

PEP is indicated for exposures classified as:

Category II: Minor bites or scratches without bleeding, or nibbles on exposed skin.

Category III: Transdermal bites or scratches, licks on broken skin, contamination of mucous membranes by saliva, or direct contact with bats.

Wound Management
Immediate and thorough wound cleansing for at least 15 minutes with soap and water or a disinfectant (e.g., povidone-iodine) is critical to reduce viral load.
Suturing is avoided unless necessary for functional or cosmetic reasons and should be delayed until rabies immunoglobulin (RIG) is administered. Highly contaminated wounds require surgical debridement and copious irrigation.

Passive and Active Immunization
Rabies Immunoglobulin (RIG): Administered once on the day of exposure (D0) along with the first vaccine dose. The RIG dose (20 IU/kg for human RIG or 40 IU/kg for purified F(ab')2 fragments) is infiltrated into and around the wound site. For mucosal exposures, RIG diluted in saline is used for rinsing.

Rabies Vaccine: A cell-culture-based vaccine is administered following either the intramuscular (IM) or

intradermal (ID) regimen.
Common schedules include:
IM: Zagreb (2-0-1-0-1) or Essen (1-1-1-1-0) over 14–28 days.
ID: Doses vary by national guidelines and patient factors.
PEP regimens are tailored for immunocompromised individuals, requiring additional vaccine doses and closer monitoring.

Additional Considerations

Antibiotic Prophylaxis: Indicated for infected or high-risk wounds using co-amoxiclav as the first-line treatment. Alternatives include co-trimoxazole and clindamycin for penicillin-allergic patients.

Tetanus Prophylaxis: Tetanus vaccination and serotherapy should be considered for patients with an uncertain or outdated immunization history.

Prevention Strategies

Pre-exposure prophylaxis (PrEP) with rabies vaccines is recommended for high-risk populations, such as individuals in endemic areas or professionals in frequent contact with animals.

Footnotes

(a) For individuals with direct exposure to bats, adhere to the specific guidelines issued by national health authorities.
(b) For HIV-positive patients, criteria include CD4 counts ≤ 25% in children under 5 years of age or less than 200 cells/mm³ in children aged 5 years and older, as well as adults.
(c) Rabies risk can be assessed either through observation of the animal (for domestic cases) or laboratory examination of the animal (if deceased). WHO advises a 10-day observation period for captured animals. If no rabies symptoms appear within this timeframe, the risk is deemed negligible, and post-exposure prophylaxis (PEP) may be stopped. For laboratory analysis of deceased animals, the head is sent to a specialized facility for confirmation. If tests are negative, PEP can be discontinued.
(d) Alternative regimens for patients allergic to penicillin:
Children: Co-trimoxazole (30 mg SMX + 6 mg TMP per kg twice daily) combined with

clindamycin (10 mg/kg three times daily).
Adults: Co-trimoxazole (800 mg SMX + 160 mg TMP twice daily) or doxycycline (100 mg twice daily or 200 mg once daily, except for pregnant and breastfeeding women) with metronidazole (500 mg three times daily).

References

1. World Health Organization. Weekly Epidemiological Record (Relevé Épidémiologique Hebdomadaire), 20 April 2018, 93rd Year, No. 16, pp. 201–220. Available at: http://apps.who.int/iris/bitstream/handle/10665/272371/WER9316.pdf?ua=1 [Accessed 25 October 2018].
2. Spencer O, Banerjee S. Animal Bites. BMJ Best Practice, 2018. [Accessed 25 October 2018].

Viral Hepatitis: Overview and Clinical Management

Viral Hepatitis: Overview and Clinical Management

Viral hepatitis refers to liver infections caused by a range of viruses, including hepatitis A, B, C, D, and E. These infections are prevalent worldwide, though the frequency varies by region. In developing countries, hepatitis A and B are more common, with most infections occurring in childhood. The clinical presentation of viral hepatitis is similar across all types, making diagnosis challenging. However, there are distinct differences in their epidemiology, immunology, and pathology, which help in distinguishing between them. Hepatitis B, C, and D can lead to chronic liver disease.

Clinical Features of Viral Hepatitis

Asymptomatic or Mild Forms: Many individuals, regardless of the viral cause, may not show symptoms or experience mild symptoms.

Icteric (Jaundice) Forms: Symptoms may develop gradually or suddenly, including fever, fatigue, nausea, gastrointestinal issues, followed by jaundice, dark urine, and light-colored stools.

Fulminant Forms: This severe form involves extensive liver cell damage and can be fatal. It is most commonly seen in individuals with hepatitis B who also have a co-infection with hepatitis D or in pregnant women infected with hepatitis E during the third trimester.

Chronic Hepatitis: Hepatitis B, C, and D can lead to long-term liver damage, cirrhosis, or liver cancer.

Transmission and Risk Groups

Hepatitis A: Primarily affects children and is transmitted through contaminated food and water (fecal-oral route). The incubation period is between 2 to 6 weeks. Hepatitis A does not lead to chronic infection.

Hepatitis B: Most commonly affects young adults and is transmitted through blood, sexual contact, or from mother to child (vertical transmission). The incubation period varies from 4 to 30 weeks, and chronicity can develop in 0.2 to 10% of cases, with some progressing to cirrhosis or liver cancer.

Hepatitis C: Also affects young adults, with transmission occurring through exposure to infected blood, including through transfusions or sexual contact. The incubation period ranges from 2 to 25 weeks, and up to 50% of cases can become chronic, leading to cirrhosis and possibly liver cancer.

Hepatitis D: This virus can only occur in people who are already infected with hepatitis B, and it is transmitted through blood and sexual contact. Chronic infection is possible, especially when hepatitis B and D co-occur, leading to rapid progression to cirrhosis.

Hepatitis E: Primarily affects young adults and is transmitted through contaminated food and water (fecal-oral). The incubation period is 2 to 8 weeks. This form is particularly dangerous for pregnant women, with a mortality rate of 20% in the third trimester.

Diagnosis and Laboratory Tests

The diagnosis of viral hepatitis is confirmed through the detection of specific antibodies or viral antigens in the blood. Hepatitis A is diagnosed by detecting IgM antibodies against the virus, while hepatitis B is identified by the presence of hepatitis B surface antigen (HBsAg) and possibly hepatitis B DNA.

Hepatitis C is diagnosed by detecting anti-HCV antibodies and HCV RNA, while hepatitis D and E are identified through similar antibody detection methods.

For chronic hepatitis cases, additional tests like elastography (Fibroscan®) are used to assess liver fibrosis, and the APRI score may help in evaluating the stage of liver disease. Liver function tests, including ALT and AST levels, and a platelet count are also important in assessing the extent of liver damage.

Treatment

Treatment aims to manage symptoms, reduce liver damage, and prevent complications like cirrhosis and liver cancer. In cases of chronic hepatitis B, antiviral drugs such as tenofovir are commonly used. For chronic hepatitis C, direct-acting antiviral drugs (e.g., sofosbuvir/velpatasvir) can lead to sustained virologic response, effectively curing the infection. For hepatitis D, the treatment is linked to managing hepatitis B, as the D virus can only exist in a host with active hepatitis B infection.

Vaccination is the primary preventive measure for hepatitis A and B. The hepatitis A vaccine is recommended for children and those at high risk, while the hepatitis B vaccine is part of routine childhood immunization. Hepatitis E has no vaccine, and preventive measures are focused on improving sanitation and hygiene.

Prevention

Individual preventive measures include vaccination (where available), safe sex practices, and avoiding contact with contaminated blood. For hepatitis B, the use of immunoglobulins after exposure can reduce the risk of infection. At the community level, promoting hygiene and sanitation, as well as screening blood for hepatitis viruses before transfusion, are crucial preventive steps.

Hepatitis remains a significant global health challenge, but advancements in treatment and prevention have made managing these infections more feasible, reducing both the spread of the disease and the risk of severe liver damage.

Footnotes

(a) For further details, please refer to the following resource: Global Dengue Transmission Map.

(b) Ensure adequate urine output, which should be at least 1 ml/kg/hour for children and 0.5 ml/kg/hour for adults. In the absence of direct measurement, confirm that the patient urinates at least every 4 hours.

(c) To prepare a 5% glucose solution in Ringer's lactate, withdraw 50 ml from a 500 ml bottle or bag of Ringer's lactate (RL), then add 50 ml of 50% glucose to the remaining 450 ml of RL, resulting in 500 ml of a 5% glucose-RL mixture.

References

1. Pan American Health Organization. Dengue: Guidelines for Patient Care in the Region of the Americas, 2nd ed. Washington, D.C.: PAHO, 2016. Available at: https://iris.paho.org/bitstream/handle/10665.2/31207/9789275118900-

eng.pdf?sequence=1&isAllowed=y [Accessed 23 Aug 2022].
2. Pan American Health Organization. Clinical Diagnosis and Treatment Guidelines for Dengue, Chikungunya, and Zika. Washington, D.C.: PAHO, 2022. Available at: https://iris.paho.org/handle/10665.2/55867 [Accessed 16 Aug 2022].

Viral Hemorrhagic Fevers (VHF)
Viral hemorrhagic fevers refer to a group of illnesses caused by different viruses with various modes of transmission. Despite their differences, these diseases share common clinical features, such as high fever and bleeding symptoms. Dengue hemorrhagic fever, which is a notable type of viral hemorrhagic fever, is discussed in detail in Chapter 8 of this book.

Clinical Features
The common syndrome observed in viral hemorrhagic fevers typically includes the following signs:
Fever exceeding 38.5°C.
Bleeding manifestations such as purpura (purple skin spots), nosebleeds (epistaxis), vomiting

blood (haematemesis), and black stools (melaena).

These clinical symptoms, although indicative of hemorrhagic fevers, are often nonspecific and can vary greatly in severity depending on the specific virus involved.

Laboratory and Geographical Aspects

A variety of viruses cause hemorrhagic fevers, with distinct reservoirs and vectors, leading to different geographic distributions:

1. Ebola and Marburg: Primarily associated with bats (as possible reservoirs), these viruses are prevalent in Africa. Infected patients require strict isolation. Clinical features often include sudden onset of malaise, vomiting, and diarrhea, with case fatality rates ranging from 60-80%.

2. Lassa Fever: Caused by rodent transmission in West Africa, Lassa fever presents with general malaise, headache, muscle pain, and facial edema. Proteinuria is commonly observed. The case fatality rate is around 15-20%.

3. Junin and Machupo Fevers: These diseases, transmitted by rodents in South America, share clinical signs such as vomiting, facial erythema, and in some cases, conjunctivitis and proteinuria, with a fatality rate of 15-30%.
4. Omsk Hemorrhagic Fever: Transmitted via ticks in Europe and Asia, this condition has a relatively low case fatality rate of 2-5%.
5. Crimean-Congo Fever: Caused by livestock and tick transmission in Africa and Asia, this fever can be fatal in 5-20% of cases and requires strict isolation measures.
6. Hantavirus (FHSR): Known to be transmitted by rodents in Asia and Europe, hantavirus presents with mild symptoms and has a case fatality rate of less than 1%.
7. Kyasanur Forest Disease: This fever, transmitted by small mammals and ticks in India, typically causes headache, muscle pain, and prostration, with a fatality rate of 2-10%.
8. Rift Valley Fever: Found in Africa and transmitted by mosquitoes, it often presents with

fever and encephalitis, leading to 30-50% fatality in certain cases.

9. Yellow Fever: Also transmitted by mosquitoes in Africa and South America, yellow fever presents with jaundice and proteinuria, and a mortality rate between 10-30%.

Diagnostic Approach

When suspecting a viral hemorrhagic fever, a sample of whole blood should be sent to a reference laboratory for serological diagnosis, along with a detailed clinical description. In situations where blood collection is difficult, filter paper can be used, though it limits the scope of testing due to the small volume of blood available.

To protect healthcare workers, personal protective equipment (PPE) such as gowns, gloves, masks, and goggles should be worn when collecting or handling samples. Proper handling involves a triple packaging system for transporting samples of Category A infectious substances.

Management

Suspicion of Viral Hemorrhagic Fever: If a patient presents with fever and hemorrhagic symptoms in an endemic region, or if there are confirmed cases of diseases such as Ebola, Marburg, Lassa, or Crimean-Congo fever, it is crucial to isolate the patient and implement strict infection control protocols.

Isolation and Treatment Protocols:

1. Isolation: Patients should be isolated in a designated area with controlled entry and exit. If necessary, barriers such as screens or partitions should be used, and only essential staff, wearing appropriate PPE, should provide care.

2. Standard Precautions: These include thorough hand washing, use of gloves when handling bodily fluids, and wearing gowns and masks during high-risk procedures. Proper disposal of medical waste and safe injection practices are essential.

3. Invasive Procedures: In the case of Ebola and Marburg, all invasive procedures, including the insertion of intravenous lines, must be performed with extreme caution as healthcare workers are at risk of contamination.

Aetiological Treatment: Ribavirin is the recommended treatment for Lassa fever and Crimean-Congo fever.

Symptomatic Treatment:

Fever management: Paracetamol is used to manage fever, while acetylsalicylic acid (aspirin) should be avoided.

Pain management: Mild pain can be managed with paracetamol, while tramadol or sublingual morphine is used for moderate to severe pain.

Hydration: Oral rehydration solutions or intravenous fluids (such as Ringer lactate) are used to manage dehydration.

Seizure management: Anticonvulsants such as benzodiazepines can be used.

Vomiting: Ondansetron can be administered to control vomiting, with specific dosages depending on the patient's age.

Vaccination:

Yellow Fever: A single dose of 0.5 ml is recommended for both children and adults. Mass vaccination campaigns are recommended during outbreaks, particularly in regions with high risk.

Rift Valley Fever: Vaccination is only recommended during an outbreak.

Infection Control and Prevention

1. Personal Protective Equipment (PPE): Before entering isolation areas, healthcare workers must wear PPE, including gloves, gowns, masks, face shields, and other protective equipment, to prevent exposure to the virus.

2. Disinfection and Safe Burial: Surfaces, clothing, and bedding should be disinfected with chlorine solutions. In case of death, the body should not be washed; instead, prompt and safe burial must take place using a body bag to minimize the risk of transmission.

References

1. World Health Organization. Clinical Management of Patients with Viral Hemorrhagic Fever: A Pocket Guide for Front-Line Health Workers. Interim emergency guidance for country adaptation, February 2016. Available at: http://apps.who.int/iris/bitstream/handle/10665/205570/978924154 49608_eng.pdf?jsessionid=15E1 7DE39631519C2051413DDCBB

C8A7?sequence=1 [Accessed 11 Jan 2019].
2. World Health Organization. Weekly Epidemiological Record, July 5, 2013, 88th Year, No. 27, 2013, 88, 269–284. Available at: https://www.who.int/wer/2013/wer8827.pdf?ua=1 [Accessed 10 Dec 2018].

HIV Infection and AIDS: Overview and Management

Human Immunodeficiency Virus (HIV) is the virus responsible for causing Acquired Immune Deficiency Syndrome (AIDS), the most severe stage of HIV infection. HIV is classified into two main subtypes: HIV-1, which is more widespread globally, and HIV-2, predominantly found in West Africa. While HIV-2 is less virulent and transmissible than HIV-1, it still contributes to the global burden of HIV/AIDS.

Pathophysiology and Evolution of HIV

HIV primarily weakens the immune system by targeting CD4 T lymphocytes, crucial cells for immune defense. As the virus progresses, CD4 counts decline, leading to increased vulnerability to infections and cancers.

Clinical Stages of HIV

The World Health Organization (WHO) classifies HIV infection into four clinical stages, which are used to assess the severity of the disease:

1. Primary HIV infection/Acute retroviral syndrome: Occurs within 2-4 weeks post-exposure. Symptoms include fever, fatigue, and lymphadenopathy, affecting 50-70% of newly infected individuals.

2. Asymptomatic HIV infection: After initial seroconversion, the patient remains asymptomatic but the virus continues to replicate, with the disease typically progressing over 10 years in developed countries.

3. Symptomatic HIV infection: As the immune system weakens, patients begin to experience more severe and frequent opportunistic infections (OIs) and other complications.

4. AIDS: Defined by a CD4 count of <200 cells/mm^3, AIDS represents the final stage where severe opportunistic infections and malignancies develop.

Laboratory Diagnosis
HIV infection is diagnosed using serological tests (detecting HIV antibodies) or virological tests (commonly used for infants). Accurate diagnosis requires at least two positive results from different test kits. Confirmatory testing is crucial to avoid false positives, especially in regions with low HIV prevalence. Testing should be voluntary, with informed consent, and follow-up counseling is necessary.

CD4 Count and Viral Load
CD4 T lymphocyte count is a key indicator of immune function. CD4 depletion predicts the likelihood of developing opportunistic infections, such as cerebral toxoplasmosis or cryptococcal meningitis, which often occur when CD4 counts fall below 100 cells/mm^3. Viral load tests are essential for monitoring HIV replication and treatment efficacy.

Opportunistic Infections
As HIV progresses, the risk of opportunistic infections (OIs) increases. In early stages, primary infections like acute retroviral syndrome are common,

but as the disease advances, more serious OIs emerge, such as tuberculosis (TB), fungal infections, and certain cancers.

1. Primary infection/acute retroviral syndrome: Develops during seroconversion, presenting with flu-like symptoms such as fever and swollen lymph nodes.
2. Asymptomatic period: Characterized by ongoing viral replication, though the patient remains without symptoms for several years.
3. Symptomatic HIV infection: The immune system's depletion leads to frequent infections and other health complications.
4. AIDS: Marked by the development of life-threatening opportunistic infections and cancers due to severe immunosuppression.

Treatment Strategies

Antiretroviral Therapy (ART) is the cornerstone of HIV management. ART, consisting of at least three medications from different classes, does not cure HIV but significantly reduces viral load, stabilizing the immune system and preventing

progression to AIDS. ART options include:
Nucleoside/nucleotide reverse transcriptase inhibitors (NRTIs), e.g., zidovudine (AZT), tenofovir (TDF).
Non-nucleoside reverse transcriptase inhibitors (NNRTIs), e.g., efavirenz (EFV).
Protease inhibitors (PIs), e.g., lopinavir (LPV).
Integrase inhibitors (IIs), e.g., dolutegravir.
The primary goal is to maintain an undetectable viral load and prevent resistance, requiring lifelong adherence to prescribed regimens. Viral load and CD4 counts should be regularly monitored to evaluate treatment effectiveness.

Prevention and Prophylaxis

Preventing HIV infection and reducing the transmission risk is crucial. Prevention methods include:
Condom use: The most effective way to prevent sexual transmission.
Male circumcision: Reduces the risk of heterosexual transmission.
Pre-exposure prophylaxis (PrEP): Antiretroviral

medications taken before exposure to HIV for individuals at high risk.

Post-exposure prophylaxis (PEP): Emergency treatment within 72 hours after potential HIV exposure.

For mother-to-child transmission (MTCT), ART during pregnancy significantly reduces the risk of vertical transmission. The Option B+ protocol, which includes lifelong ART for HIV-positive pregnant women, is globally recommended.

Opportunistic Infection Prevention and Management

Without ART, individuals with HIV inevitably progress to AIDS. However, primary prophylaxis with antibiotics like co-trimoxazole is essential to prevent infections like pneumocystis and toxoplasmosis in patients with low CD4 counts. Secondary prophylaxis is also critical for those who have already developed specific opportunistic infections, aiming to prevent their recurrence.

Example of Prophylactic Treatments:

Co-trimoxazole: Used to prevent infections like pneumocystis pneumonia (PCP) and toxoplasmosis in patients with CD4 counts below 200 cells/mm^3.
Fluconazole: For cryptococcal meningitis.
Itraconazole: Used for fungal infections like histoplasmosis.
Special Considerations
Pain Management:
Chronic pain, often associated with opportunistic infections and immune suppression, should be managed using appropriate analgesics as outlined in clinical pain management protocols.
Conclusion
The management of HIV requires comprehensive care, including early diagnosis, ART, prophylactic treatments, and careful monitoring of immune status. Preventive measures, especially in high-risk populations, are key to reducing the spread of HIV. Through ongoing medical advancements and adherence to ART regimens, individuals living with HIV can lead long and healthy lives, though lifelong treatment is

essential. Regular monitoring, including viral load and CD4 count, ensures that any complications or opportunistic infections are identified and managed promptly.

Footnotes

(a) For further details, see: World Health Organization. Antiretroviral Medications for HIV Treatment and Prevention: Public Health Guidelines, 2nd edition. Geneva: World Health Organization, 2016. Available at WHO link.

References

1. World Health Organization. Case Definitions for HIV Surveillance and Updated Clinical Staging and Immunological Classification of HIV-Related Disease in Adults and Children, 2007. Available at WHO link [Accessed May 17, 2018].

2. World Health Organization. Guidelines for the Diagnosis, Prevention, and Management of Cryptococcal Disease in HIV-Infected Adults, Adolescents, and Children, Geneva, 2018. Available at WHO link [Accessed May 17, 2018].

Chapter 9
Genito-Urinary Diseases

This chapter covers a range of genito-urinary conditions, including:

Nephrotic Syndrome in Children: A disorder characterized by protein loss in the urine, leading to swelling and other complications.

Urolithiasis: The formation of stones in the urinary tract, causing pain and urinary symptoms.

Acute Cystitis: An infection of the bladder, typically causing painful urination and frequent urges to urinate.

Acute Pyelonephritis: A kidney infection that may present with fever, flank pain, and urinary symptoms.

Acute Prostatitis: An infection of the prostate gland, often associated with pain, fever, and urinary difficulties.

Genital Infections: Includes a variety of bacterial, viral, and fungal infections affecting the genital region.

Urethral Discharge: A common symptom of infections or inflammation in the urethra.

Abnormal Vaginal Discharge: Changes in vaginal discharge that can indicate infection or other reproductive health issues.
Genital Ulcers: Painful sores that may be caused by infections like herpes or syphilis.
Lower Abdominal Pain in Women: Pain localized in the lower abdomen, often related to reproductive organs.
Upper Genital Tract Infections (UGTI): Infections that affect the upper reproductive organs, such as the uterus and fallopian tubes.
Venereal Warts: Caused by human papillomavirus (HPV), these are growths or lumps that appear on the genital area.
Major Genital Infections (Summary): A brief overview of significant infections affecting the genital region.
Abnormal Uterine Bleeding (in the absence of pregnancy): Irregular bleeding from the uterus, often linked to hormonal imbalances or structural abnormalities.
Nephrotic Syndrome in Children
Nephrotic syndrome (NS) in children is defined by the presence of edema, significant

proteinuria, low serum albumin, and elevated lipid levels. It can be classified into:

Primary (Idiopathic) Nephrotic Syndrome: The most common form in children aged 1-10 years, typically responsive to corticosteroid therapy.

Secondary Nephrotic Syndrome: Often linked to systemic infections such as post-infectious glomerulonephritis, hepatitis B and C, HIV, malaria, and schistosomiasis. Treatment of the underlying infection can resolve the condition.

Children with NS face an increased risk of complications, including thromboembolism, bacterial infections (especially from Streptococcus pneumoniae), and malnutrition. Without treatment, the condition can progress to renal failure.

Clinical Presentation

Patients typically present with soft, pitting edema, which is more pronounced in the morning around the face and eyes and tends to shift to the legs as the day progresses. This edema may eventually become generalized, affecting the abdomen (ascites) and chest (pleural effusions). Differentiation from edema seen in severe acute malnutrition (SAM) is crucial; in SAM, edema is typically bilateral and non-variable with body position, extending to the hands and face in severe cases.

Diagnostic Criteria

To diagnose primary NS, two key conditions must be met:

1. Heavy Proteinuria: Confirmed by dipstick urine tests, showing protein levels of +++ or ≥300 mg/dl.

2. Absence of Secondary Infections: Conditions such as hepatitis, HIV, malaria, and schistosomiasis must be ruled out (refer to Chapter 8 for more on these infections).

Laboratory Findings

Urine: Protein levels in NS are ≥300 mg/dl or 30 g/liter. If there is also macroscopic or microscopic hematuria, further investigation for glomerulonephritis is warranted.

Blood Tests: Low serum albumin (<30 g/liter) and elevated lipids are typical. Blood urea nitrogen (BUN) and creatinine are usually normal unless renal function is impaired.

Management

Corticosteroid Therapy: Prednisolone or prednisone is the first-line treatment for primary NS.

Infections: Before initiating corticosteroids, treat any underlying infections such as pneumonia, peritonitis, or sepsis. Exclude active tuberculosis and, if necessary, begin antituberculous treatment.

Diet and Fluid Management

Diet: A no-salt-added diet is recommended to help manage edema.

Fluid Intake: Fluids should not be restricted unless there is severe edema, in which case fluid intake may be limited to 75% of normal while closely monitoring urine output.

Activity: Encourage physical activity to reduce the risk of thromboembolism.

Follow-up Care

Discharge: Once the child's condition stabilizes, discharge is appropriate with monthly follow-ups (or more frequently as needed) for weight and urine monitoring.

Parent Education: Instruct parents to continue the no-salt-added diet and seek medical attention if signs of infection or thromboembolism occur.

Infection Prevention and Immunization

Ensure the child is up-to-date with recommended vaccinations:

Under 5 years: Haemophilus influenzae type B, pneumococcal, and meningococcal A conjugate vaccines.

Over 5 years: Tetanus, measles, pneumococcal, and meningococcal A conjugate vaccines.

Management of Intravascular Volume Depletion

If signs of shock (e.g., decreased urine output, poor capillary refill, cold extremities) are present, administer human albumin IV (1 g/kg), or if unavailable, use Ringer lactate or sodium chloride. Diuretics such as furosemide should only be used if hypovolemia is corrected, with close monitoring for dehydration and electrolyte imbalances.

Specialized Treatment for Steroid-Resistant NS

In cases where the NS is resistant to steroids, further specialized treatment, including possible renal biopsy, is needed. As a last resort, enalapril (0.1 to 0.3 mg/kg) may help reduce proteinuria and delay renal failure, though the prognosis remains poor without specialized care.

Complications

Severe Edema-Related Respiratory Distress: This can occur in very young children or those with steroid-resistant NS. Management requires urgent intervention.

Footnote

Nephrotic-range proteinuria in children is defined as urinary protein excretion greater than 50 mg/kg daily. If a 24-hour urine collection is not feasible, a urine dipstick can serve as an alternative for monitoring protein levels.

Urolithiasis

Overview

Urolithiasis refers to the formation and passage of calculi (stones) within the urinary tract.

While most calculi pass spontaneously, complications can arise if there is significant renal dysfunction or secondary infection. In such cases, surgical referral should be considered.

Clinical Features

Many urinary stones do not produce symptoms and may only be discovered incidentally during radiologic examinations. Symptoms typically occur when stones cause partial or complete obstruction or lead to infection. Key clinical manifestations include:

Renal Colic: Intermittent, severe flank to pelvic pain that often radiates, associated with nausea and vomiting. The pain can lead to restlessness, with patients unable to find a comfortable position.

Haematuria: Blood in the urine, possibly with visible gravel or stones.

Secondary Infection: If infection develops, fever and signs of pyelonephritis may be present.

Management

Encourage patients to increase fluid intake to promote stone passage. For pain relief, administer analgesics according to the severity (refer to Chapter 1 for pain management). If secondary infection is suspected, treat with antibiotics appropriate for pyelonephritis.

In cases where renal dysfunction or infection does not improve with conservative measures, surgical referral should be considered

Acute Cystitis

Overview

Acute cystitis is a bladder and urethral infection most commonly affecting women and girls over the age of 2. The condition is frequently caused by Escherichia coli (70% of cases), although other pathogens like Proteus mirabilis, Enterococcus sp., Klebsiella sp., and Staphylococcus saprophyticus (especially in young women) are also implicated.

Clinical Features

The primary symptoms include:

Dysuria: A painful or burning sensation while urinating.

Increased Urgency and Frequency: An urgent need to urinate, often with small volumes of urine.

In Children: Crying or discomfort during urination; occasional involuntary urination.

Absence of Systemic Symptoms: Typically, there is no fever or flank pain, and systemic signs such as chills or fatigue are absent.

It is crucial to distinguish cystitis from pyelonephritis, which may present with fever and flank pain.

Investigations

A dipstick urinalysis is often sufficient for diagnosis. Look for:

Nitrites: Indicative of the presence of enterobacteria.

Leukocytes: Suggestive of inflammation or infection in the urinary tract.

If the dipstick test shows positive results for nitrites or leukocytes, empiric antibiotic therapy should be initiated. However, in regions where urinary schistosomiasis is endemic, consider testing for Schistosoma if hematuria is present, particularly in children aged 5-15 years.

In cases where urine microscopy is available, confirmatory testing can be done to identify the causative pathogen.

Treatment
Treatment for cystitis varies by age and condition:
In Girls ≥2 years:
Cefixime (8 mg/kg once daily for 3 days)
Amoxicillin/Clavulanic acid (12.5 mg/kg twice daily for 3 days)
In Nonpregnant Young Women:
Fosfomycin-trometamol (3 g single dose)
Nitrofurantoin (100 mg thrice daily for 5 days)
In Pregnant or Lactating Women:
Fosfomycin-trometamol (3 g single dose)
Nitrofurantoin (100 mg thrice daily for 7 days, not in last month of pregnancy)
Cefixime (200 mg twice daily for 5 days)
If symptoms persist despite treatment, or if recurrent cystitis occurs (more than 3-4 episodes per year), consider additional investigations to rule out underlying conditions such as bladder stones, urinary tuberculosis, or gonorrhea. In the case of treatment failure, Ciprofloxacin (500 mg twice

daily for 3 days) may be appropriate for short courses.

Special Considerations

For patients with recurrent cystitis, additional diagnostic testing such as POCUS (Point-of-care Ultrasound) should be conducted to evaluate for urinary tract abnormalities, including bladder stones or other pathologies. However, POCUS should only be performed by trained clinicians.

Conclusion

Urolithiasis and cystitis are common urinary tract conditions that require prompt recognition and appropriate treatment. Fluid intake, analgesia, and antibiotics are cornerstone treatments, but surgical intervention may be necessary in cases of complicated urolithiasis. Monitoring for recurrent infections and complications is critical in managing these conditions effectively.

Footnote

(a) Point-of-care ultrasound (POCUS) should only be conducted and analyzed by healthcare professionals with appropriate training and expertise.

Acute Pyelonephritis

Acute pyelonephritis is an infection of the renal parenchyma, more prevalent in women than men. It is commonly caused by the same pathogens responsible for cystitis (see Acute Cystitis, Chapter 9). Pyelonephritis can be severe, especially in pregnant women, neonates, and infants. The management approach depends on the severity of symptoms, the presence of complications, or the risk of complications.

Clinical Features:

Neonates and Infants:

A urinary tract infection (UTI) should be suspected in any neonate or infant presenting with unexplained fever or signs of septic syndrome without a clear source of infection.

Older Children and Adults:

Symptoms include fever, irritability, vomiting, poor feeding, and abdominal tenderness, particularly upon palpation of the lower abdomen. Fever is a key sign but its absence does not rule out

pyelonephritis. In some cases, fever may be the only symptom, especially in children and neonates.
Common signs include unilateral flank pain or abdominal tenderness, nausea, vomiting, and, in more severe cases, fever >38°C.
Laboratory Findings:
See Acute Cystitis, Chapter 9 for specific laboratory tests.
Criteria for Hospital Admission:
At-risk groups include children, pregnant women, men, individuals with structural or functional urinary tract abnormalities (e.g., stones, malformations), and patients with severe immunodeficiency.
Complicated pyelonephritis may involve urinary tract obstruction, renal abscess, or emphysematous pyelonephritis, particularly in diabetic patients.
Severe infection signs include sepsis (infection with organ dysfunction), septic shock, dehydration, or vomiting preventing hydration and oral antibiotic administration.
If there is no clinical improvement within 24 hours of

starting oral antibiotics in women treated as outpatients, hospitalization may be required.
Treatment:
Children under One Month:
Ampicillin IV (slow infusion):
For neonates <2 kg: 50 mg/kg every 12 hours for 7–10 days.
For neonates ≥2 kg: 50 mg/kg every 8 hours for 7–10 days.
Gentamicin IV (slow infusion):
For neonates <2 kg: 3 mg/kg daily for 5 days.
For neonates ≥2 kg: 5 mg/kg daily for 5 days.
Alternative: Cefotaxime IV for 7–10 days at appropriate dosages based on age and weight.
Children 1 Month and Older:
Ceftriaxone IM or IV (slow infusion): 50 mg/kg once daily until the child's condition improves (minimum of 3 days), then switch to oral antibiotics:
Amoxicillin/Clavulanic acid PO:
Children <40 kg: 25 mg/kg twice daily for 10–14 days.
For children ≥40 kg: Amoxicillin/Clavulanic acid at 2000 mg daily (two 500/62.5 mg tablets twice daily).
Adults:
Uncomplicated Pyelonephritis:

Ceftriaxone IM (single dose): 1 g or Gentamicin IM (single dose): 5 mg/kg.

Follow-up with Ciprofloxacin PO: 500 mg twice daily for 7 days, or Amoxicillin/Clavulanic acid PO (2000 mg daily) for 10–14 days, or Cefixime PO: 200 mg twice daily for 10–14 days.

Complicated Pyelonephritis:
Ampicillin IV (slow infusion): 2 g every 6 hours for at least 3 days + Gentamicin IM: 5 mg/kg daily for 3 days.

Alternatively, use Ceftriaxone IV (1 g once daily) for at least 3 days + Gentamicin IM for 3 days in cases of sepsis.

Follow up with Amoxicillin/Clavulanic acid PO or another antibiotic based on susceptibility for 10–14 days.

Additional Management:
Fever and Pain: Avoid NSAIDs (see Fever, Chapter 1).

Hydration: Ensure adequate fluid intake (1.5 liters daily in adults), particularly in children who are at greater risk of dehydration. Treat dehydration as needed (see Dehydration, Chapter 1).

Septic Shock: Manage septic shock as necessary.

Footnotes:
(a) Pyelonephritis is uncommon in men, and bacterial prostatitis should be considered in febrile urinary tract infections in men.
(b) The solvent for IM ceftriaxone contains lidocaine. Ceftriaxone reconstituted with this solvent should never be administered intravenously. For IV administration, use only water for injection.

References:
Gupta K, Hooton TM, Naber KG, Wullt B, Colgan R, Miller LG, Moran GJ, Nicolle LE, Raz R, Schaeffer AJ, Soper DE, Infectious Diseases Society of America, European Society for Microbiology and Infectious Diseases. "International clinical practice guidelines for the treatment of acute uncomplicated cystitis and pyelonephritis in women: A 2010 update." Clin Infect Dis. 2011;52(5):e103.

Acute Prostatitis: A Comprehensive Overview

Definition

Acute prostatitis is a bacterial infection of the prostate gland. Escherichia coli is the most common pathogen, though other bacteria such as Proteus mirabilis, Klebsiella sp., Pseudomonas aeruginosa, and Enterococcus sp. have also been identified. If not effectively treated, acute prostatitis may progress to chronic prostatitis.

Clinical Features

Common signs and symptoms of acute prostatitis include:

Fever and chills: Often severe, indicating systemic infection.

Lower urinary tract symptoms: These include dysuria (painful urination), frequency, and urgency, which are commonly associated with cystitis.

Pain: This can occur in the perineum, urethra, penis, or rectum.

Urinary retention: Difficulty or inability to urinate due to prostate swelling.

Digital rectal examination (DRE): Typically, a very painful procedure, and may reveal a fluctuating mass, suggesting a prostatic abscess.

Urinalysis: Findings often include leukocyturia (white blood cells in urine), pyuria (pus in urine), and possibly visible hematuria (blood in urine).

Diagnosis and Management

Antibiotic Therapy:
Empiric antibiotic treatment is initiated to target the most likely pathogens.
A typical regimen involves ciprofloxacin 500 mg orally twice daily for 14 days. If symptoms resolve, the treatment is discontinued after this period. If symptoms persist, the course is extended for an additional 14 days.

Symptomatic Treatment:
Hydration: Ensure the patient is well-hydrated (approximately 1.5 liters of fluid daily).
Pain and Fever Management: Medications such as NSAIDs can be used to manage pain and reduce fever.
Referral: In cases where a prostatic abscess is suspected, referral to a surgeon is necessary for drainage.

References

National Institute for Health and Care Excellence (NICE) guidelines on prostatitis (acute): antimicrobial prescribing, updated August 2021.
Genital Infections: Management and Syndromic Approach

Challenges in Diagnosis and Treatment

Genital infections (GIs) present unique diagnostic challenges, including:

Non-specific symptoms: Many genital infections are asymptomatic, and when symptoms are present, they are often nonspecific.

Laboratory Limitations: Field testing is not always reliable, and many infections may not be easily identified.

Mixed Infections: Co-infections with multiple pathogens are common.

HIV-Infected Patients: These individuals are at a higher risk of treatment failure or recurrence.

To address these challenges, the World Health Organization (WHO) recommends syndromic management, which involves treating based on clinical syndromes rather than waiting for laboratory results. This approach simplifies treatment in resource-limited settings.

Basic Principles of GI Management

Early Treatment: Treatment should begin at the first point of contact with healthcare providers. Delaying treatment for diagnostic results can worsen the infection and increase transmission risk.

Partner Treatment: In cases of sexually transmitted infections (STIs), the sexual partner should be treated simultaneously to prevent reinfection.

Single-Dose Regimens: Preferred for many common infections (e.g., azithromycin for chlamydia, ceftriaxone for gonorrhea).

Prevention and Education: Education on STIs, safe sex practices, and HIV testing should be provided.

Special Situation: Sexual Violence

In the context of sexual violence, the approach goes beyond diagnosing and treating infections:

Comprehensive Care: Includes physical examination, lab tests (if available), and providing immediate medical care.

Mental Health Support: Psychological care is essential for addressing trauma-related mental health issues, such as anxiety, depression, and PTSD.

Prophylactic and Curative Treatment:

HIV Prophylaxis: Initiate antiretroviral therapy as soon as possible if within 48-72 hours after exposure.

Emergency Contraception: Administer within 72 hours to prevent pregnancy.

STI Prevention: Treat with a single dose of azithromycin and ceftriaxone, or alternatives if unavailable.

Vaccination: Hepatitis B vaccination and tetanus prophylaxis should also be considered.

Urethral Discharge: Diagnosis and Treatment

Overview

Urethral discharge is primarily seen in males and is commonly caused by Neisseria gonorrhoeae (gonorrhea) and Chlamydia trachomatis (chlamydia). Symptoms include dysuria and urethral discharge, and in the absence of visible discharge, the urethra should be gently milked to confirm the diagnosis.

Diagnosis

Clinical Examination: A urethral smear can help identify gonococci (Gram-negative intracellular diplococci) through Gram staining.

Empiric Treatment: In the absence of rapid diagnostic tests, treat empirically for both gonorrhea and chlamydia, especially when laboratory confirmation is not possible.

Management

Treatment for Chlamydia: Azithromycin 1g orally in a single dose, or doxycycline 100 mg twice daily for 7 days.

Treatment for Gonorrhea: Ceftriaxone 500 mg IM in a single dose, or cefixime 400 mg orally in a single dose.

Partner Treatment

The sexual partner should receive the same treatment, regardless of whether symptoms are present.

Abnormal Vaginal Discharge: A Detailed Clinical Overview

Abnormal vaginal discharge is characterized by changes in the usual discharge in terms of color, consistency, or odor. This can include discolored, purulent, or foul-smelling discharge. It is frequently accompanied by symptoms such as vulvar itching, pain during intercourse (dyspareunia), painful or difficult urination (dysuria), or lower abdominal pain. Women presenting with these symptoms should undergo a thorough evaluation to detect any abnormal discharge.

Abnormal discharge may be indicative of an infection affecting the vagina (vaginitis), cervix (cervicitis), or upper genital tract. Accurate clinical diagnosis requires careful inspection of the vulva and a speculum exam to assess for signs of cervical or vaginal inflammation and discharge. Additionally, a bimanual pelvic examination should be performed to rule out any upper genital tract infection, particularly when the patient presents with lower abdominal pain or cervical motion tenderness.

Common Causative Organisms:

1. Vaginitis: The primary pathogens include Gardnerella vaginalis (bacterial vaginosis), Trichomonas vaginalis

(trichomoniasis), and Candida albicans (candidiasis).

2. Cervicitis: The most common pathogens responsible are Neisseria gonorrhoeae (gonorrhea) and Chlamydia trachomatis (chlamydia).

3. Upper Genital Tract Infections: Infections of the upper genital tract should be considered in cases where symptoms indicate further complications.

Case Management and Laboratory Investigation:

Vaginitis: Diagnosis involves identifying the specific pathogen through clinical examination and laboratory tests, such as wet mount microscopy, PCR-based assays, or Gram stains.

Cervicitis: This condition may be difficult to diagnose, and in uncertain cases, it is advisable to initiate treatment targeting both Chlamydia trachomatis and Neisseria gonorrhoeae.

Routine testing for both pathogens is recommended, especially when the patient presents with risk factors such as a new sexual partner, multiple partners, or a history of sexual

violence. For diagnostic accuracy, molecular (PCR) tests like Xpert molecular testing for C. trachomatis and N. gonorrhoeae are preferred.
Microscopic examination of a fresh wet smear can reveal:
Trichomonas vaginalis (mobile trophozoites) in trichomoniasis
Yeast cells and hyphae in candidiasis
Clue cells in bacterial vaginosis
Treatment Protocol:
1. Chlamydia Treatment:
Non-pregnant women:
Azithromycin 1 g orally as a single dose, or
Doxycycline 100 mg orally twice daily for 7 days
Pregnant women:
Azithromycin 1 g orally as a single dose, or
Erythromycin 500 mg orally 4 times daily for 7 days
Ceftriaxone 500 mg IM (single dose) or Cefixime 400 mg orally (single dose)
2. Gonorrhea Treatment:
Non-pregnant women:
Ceftriaxone 500 mg IM (single dose) or Cefixime 400 mg orally (single dose)
Pregnant women:

Ceftriaxone 500 mg IM (single dose) or Cefixime 400 mg orally (single dose)
3. Bacterial Vaginosis and Trichomoniasis:
Tinidazole 2 g orally as a single dose, or
Metronidazole 2 g orally as a single dose
In the case of treatment failure, tinidazole 500 mg orally twice daily for 5 days, or metronidazole 400–500 mg twice daily for 7 days
4. Vulvovaginal Candidiasis:
Clotrimazole 500 mg vaginal tablet, 1 tablet inserted at bedtime, as a single dose
If extensive vulvar involvement is present, combine with miconazole 2% cream applied twice daily for 7 days.
Partner Treatment:
In cases of vaginitis or cervicitis, sexual partners should be treated with the same regimen as the patient, even if asymptomatic. For vulvovaginal candidiasis, partner treatment is only necessary if symptoms such as itching and redness of the glans or prepuce are present.

Genital Ulcers: Clinical Approach

Genital ulcers refer to vesicular, ulcerative, or erosive lesions in the genital area, which may be accompanied by inguinal lymphadenopathy. These lesions may be indicative of sexually transmitted infections (STIs). The primary pathogens responsible for genital ulcers include Treponema pallidum (syphilis), Haemophilus (chancroid), Herpes simplex virus (genital herpes), and Chlamydia trachomatis (lymphogranuloma).

Case Management and Laboratory Investigations:

Syphilis: Laboratory tests such as rapid plasma reagin (RPR) or VDRL may not always provide definitive results, especially in early primary syphilis.

Chancroid: Diagnosis can be confirmed through PCR testing and bacterial culture.

Treatment of Genital Ulcers:

1. Genital Herpes:

First episode: Acyclovir 400 mg orally three times daily for 7 days.

Recurrent episodes: Acyclovir 400 mg orally three times daily for 5 days.

For patients with frequent recurrences (more than 6 episodes annually), additional management for HIV may be considered.

2. Syphilis:

Early syphilis: Benzathine benzylpenicillin 2.4 MIU I'M in a single dose.

Late latent syphilis: Benzathine benzylpenicillin 2.4 MUI I'M weekly for 3 weeks.

For penicillin-allergic patients: Doxycycline 100 mg orally twice daily for 14 days or erythromycin 500 mg orally four times daily for 14 days.

3. Chancroid:

Azithromycin 1 g orally as a single dose, or

Ceftriaxone 250 mg IM as a single dose.

Erythromycin 500 mg orally four times daily for 7 days is also an alternative.

4. Lymphogranuloma Venereum:

Erythromycin 500 mg orally four times daily for 14 days, or

Doxycycline 100 mg orally twice daily for 14 days.

5. Donovanosis:
Azithromycin 1 g on day 1, followed by 500 mg daily until lesion resolution.
In HIV-positive patients, add gentamicin IM 6 mg/kg once daily.

Partner Treatment:
The sexual partner should receive the same treatment as the patient, regardless of symptoms, except in the case of genital herpes, where treatment is only necessary if the partner is symptomatic.

References:
1. Centers for Disease Control and Prevention. Syphilis Pocket Guide for Providers. 2017. Link
2. World Health Organization. WHO Guidelines for the Treatment of Treponema pallidum (Syphilis), 2016. Link

Lower Abdominal Pain in Women: Diagnosis and Management

When a woman presents with lower abdominal pain, it is essential to consider potential upper genital tract infections (UGTIs), which include endometritis and salpingitis, both of which may lead to complications such as peritonitis, pelvic abscesses, or septicemia. A thorough gynecological examination is crucial in such cases.

Diagnostic Approach:

Point-of-Care Ultrasound (POCUS): If available, POCUS should be used to perform a FAST (Focused Assessment with Sonography for Trauma) exam to check for free fluid or urological abnormalities. Additionally, pelvic views can help identify uterine or adnexal pathologies. Consulting a gynecologist, either locally or through telemedicine services, is recommended for a comprehensive evaluation.

Clinical Examination:

Vulvar Inspection and Speculum Examination: Check for any purulent discharge or signs of inflammation.

Abdominal and Bimanual Pelvic Exam: Assess for tenderness on cervical motion or any abnormal masses.

Case Management: For UGTIs, antibiotic treatment is tailored to the suspected pathogens. In cases where peritonitis or a pelvic abscess is suspected, a surgical consultation should be sought while initiating empirical antibiotic therapy.

Upper Genital Tract Infections (UGTI)

UGTIs are infections of the uterus (endometritis) and/or the fallopian tubes (salpingitis). They can result from sexually transmitted infections or occur post-childbirth or abortion.

Clinical Features: Infections may manifest with abdominal pain, abnormal vaginal discharge, fever, dyspareunia, and dysuria. Cervical motion tenderness, adnexal tenderness, and an abdominal mass are key clinical signs.

Management: Antibiotic therapy should cover the most common pathogens, including Neisseria gonorrhoeae, Chlamydia trachomatis, and anaerobes. The treatment regimen often involves:

Ambulatory Treatment:

Cefixime 400 mg orally in a single dose, or ceftriaxone 500 mg intramuscularly (IM) in a single dose.

Doxycycline 100 mg orally twice daily for 14 days.

Metronidazole 500 mg orally twice daily for 14 days.
Hospital Treatment:
Ceftriaxone 1 g IM or IV daily.
Doxycycline 100 mg twice daily for 14 days.
Metronidazole 500 mg twice daily for 14 days. Continue antibiotics for 24–48 hours after symptoms improve, then switch to doxycycline (or erythromycin) and metronidazole to complete a 14-day course.
If the patient has an intrauterine device (IUD) in place, removal is recommended.

Venereal Warts (Genital Warts)
Venereal warts are benign growths caused by the human papillomavirus (HPV). These warts can appear as raised, painless lumps that may cluster or have a cauliflower-like appearance.

Treatment Options:
For External Warts < 3 cm and Vaginal Warts:
Podophyllotoxin 0.5% solution can be self-applied for external warts or applied by a healthcare provider for vaginal warts. The solution should be applied twice daily for up to 4 weeks.

For Warts > 3 cm or in Sensitive Areas (Cervix, Urethra, Rectum, Pregnancy):
Surgical excision, cryotherapy, or electrocoagulation may be necessary.
Sexually Transmitted Infections (STIs) and Treatment Regimen
Gonorrhea (Neisseria gonorrhoeae):
Clinical features include vaginal discharge, cervicitis, dysuria, and UGTI. The diagnosis is confirmed via PCR, or a Gram stain revealing intracellular diplococci.
Treatment: Ceftriaxone 500 mg IM as a single dose, plus azithromycin 1 g orally as a single dose. Treat for Chlamydia trachomatis concurrently.
Chlamydia (Chlamydia trachomatis):
Often asymptomatic, but can cause cervicitis and UGTIs. Diagnosed via PCR.
Treatment: Azithromycin 1 g orally as a single dose or doxycycline 200 mg daily for 7 days. Treatment for gonorrhea should also be considered if Neisseria gonorrhoeae is suspected.

Trichomoniasis (Trichomonas vaginalis):
Symptoms include yellow-green vaginal discharge and vulvar irritation. The infection can also be asymptomatic in men.
Treatment: Tinidazole or metronidazole 2 g orally as a single dose.
Bacterial Vaginosis (Gardnerella vaginalis):
Characterized by a homogenous, gray-white discharge with a fishy odor, a pH >4.5, and the presence of clue cells on wet mount or Gram stain.
Treatment: Metronidazole or tinidazole 2 g orally as a single dose.
Candidiasis (Candida albicans):
Pruritus and vulvovaginitis, with a creamy discharge, are common symptoms.
Treatment: Antifungal therapy (e.g., fluconazole or topical agents).
In all cases, follow-up care should include reassessment of the patient's condition to ensure appropriate response to therapy and management of complications.

Management of Abnormal Uterine Bleeding (Non-Pregnancy-Related)

Last updated: October 2021

For the management of bleeding during pregnancy, refer to the guide "Essential Obstetric and Newborn Care," MSF.

General Approach:

In women of reproductive age, the first step in assessing abnormal uterine bleeding is to determine whether the bleeding is related to pregnancy. A pregnancy test should be conducted to rule out this possibility.

Initial Assessment:

1. Rapid Evaluation of Bleeding Severity: It is crucial to assess how severe the bleeding is to guide further interventions.

2. Pelvic Examination:

Speculum Examination: Identify the bleeding's origin—whether it is from the vagina, cervix, or uterine cavity. Evaluate the appearance of the cervix and quantify the intensity of bleeding.

Bimanual Examination: Check for cervical motion tenderness, uterine enlargement, or

irregularities, which may indicate underlying pathology.
3. Additional History: Assess for recent trauma or surgical interventions that could be related to the bleeding.
4. Laboratory Investigations: Measure hemoglobin levels to assess and manage potential anemia.
If signs of shock are present, refer to Chapter 1: Shock for further management.
Management of Heavy Bleeding:
Initial Treatment:
Begin an IV infusion of Ringer's lactate to maintain circulatory volume.
Continuously monitor vital signs, especially heart rate and blood pressure.
Pharmacological Intervention:
Administer Tranexamic acid (IV): 10 mg/kg (max. 600 mg) every 8 hours. After bleeding is controlled, switch to oral Tranexamic acid: 1 g three times a day for up to five days.
If bleeding persists or there is a contraindication to Tranexamic acid, consider alternative treatments:

Ethinylestradiol/Levonorgestrel (Oral): 0.03 mg/0.15 mg tablet, one tablet three times daily for 7 days.

Medroxyprogesterone acetate (Oral): 20 mg, three times daily for 7 days.

Severe Bleeding and Surgical Options:

In cases of massive hemorrhage or failure to respond to medical treatment, surgical options should be considered:

Surgical Management: Procedures such as dilation and curettage, intrauterine balloon placement, or, as a last resort, hysterectomy.

If the patient needs to be transferred to a surgical facility, prepare for potential transport challenges, ensuring the patient has an IV line and, if possible, family members who can act as blood donors.

Point-of-Care Ultrasound (POCUS):

If available, perform Focused Assessment with Sonography for Trauma (FAST) to detect free fluid and evaluate for urological abnormalities.

Perform pelvic views to identify potential uterine or adnexal pathology.

Differential Diagnosis:

1. Cervical Cancer: A friable, hard, ulcerated, or hypertrophic mass on the cervix may indicate cervical cancer. Surgical treatment, chemotherapy, radiation therapy, or palliative care is required based on the cancer's stage. While awaiting definitive treatment, tranexamic acid (oral) can be used to reduce bleeding (1 g three times daily for up to five days).

2. Cervicitis or Pelvic Inflammatory Disease: In cases of light or moderate bleeding with purulent discharge and pelvic pain, consider cervicitis or salpingitis. Diagnosis and treatment should be guided by clinical findings and further investigations (refer to Chapter on abnormal vaginal discharge and upper genital tract infections).

3. Uterine Fibroids: An enlarged, irregular uterus may suggest uterine fibroids. If medical management fails, surgical options are necessary. If surgery

is not feasible, treat it as functional uterine bleeding.

4. Functional Uterine Bleeding: In the absence of other findings (normal uterus and cervix), functional uterine bleeding is a possible diagnosis. For initial treatment, use oral Tranexamic acid as previously described. In cases of recurrent bleeding, it may be combined with NSAIDs (e.g., ibuprofen, 3 to 5 days), and long-term treatments may include:

Levonorgestrel Intrauterine Device (IUD).

Ethinylestradiol/Levonorgestrel (Oral): One tablet daily.

Medroxyprogesterone acetate (IM): 150 mg every 3 months.

Medroxyprogesterone acetate (Oral): 10–30 mg daily for 21 days, repeating monthly.

Note: Always rule out other causes of bleeding, such as poorly tolerated contraceptives, endometrial cancer in postmenopausal women, or genitourinary schistosomiasis (in endemic areas).

Footnotes

(a) POCUS should only be performed and interpreted by

clinicians with appropriate training.
(b) The drug mentioned above does not have contraceptive effects.

References

American College of Obstetricians and Gynecologists. Management of acute abnormal uterine bleeding in nonpregnant reproductive-aged women. Obstet Gynecol. 2013 Apr;121(4):891-6. Available at: ACOG website.

Chapter 10
Medical and Minor Surgical Procedures

This chapter covers a range of medical and minor surgical procedures for managing common conditions:

1. Dressings: Techniques for properly dressing wounds to promote healing and prevent infection.

2. Treatment of Simple Wounds: Guidelines for cleaning and treating minor wounds to minimize complications.

3. Burns: Management strategies for burns, including classification and appropriate treatment.

4. Cutaneous Abscess: Approaches for draining and managing skin abscesses to prevent spread of infection.
5. Pyomyositis: Treatment of bacterial infections in muscle tissue, typically requiring drainage and antibiotics.
6. Leg Ulcers: Care strategies for managing chronic or acute leg ulcers to promote healing and reduce infection risks.
7. Necrotizing Infections of the Skin and Soft Tissues: Urgent intervention for severe infections leading to tissue death, requiring surgical debridement and antibiotics.
8. Venomous Bites and Stings: Management of bites and stings from venomous animals, including antivenom use and supportive care.
9. Dental Infections: Approaches to treating infections within the mouth, including abscesses and gum infections.

Dressing Wounds: A Comprehensive Approach

The main objective when dressing wounds is to facilitate optimal healing while minimizing the risk of infection.

This involves cleaning, disinfecting, and protecting the wound while adhering to strict hygiene protocols.

Not all wounds require dressings. For example, a clean, sutured wound that has been properly closed for several days or a small dry wound may not need dressing.

Equipment Needed for Dressing

1. Sterile Instruments

Instruments used for dressing a single patient's wound should be sterilized together in a sterile wrapping, such as paper or fabric, or a metallic box. The set may include 5 to 10 compresses. If sterile instruments are unavailable, sterile gloves can be used for the procedure.

2. Renewable Supplies

Proper care organization is crucial to maintaining asepsis and preventing contamination between patients. Essential tools include:

Forceps (Kocher or Pean)

Surgical scissors or scalpel for excising necrotic tissue or cutting gauze and sutures

Sterile compresses

Non-sterile gloves for handling

Adhesive tape or gauze bandages
Sterile sodium chloride (0.9%) or sterile water
Antiseptics (such as povidone-iodine or paraffin compresses)
Analgesics (if necessary)

3. Organizing the Care Space

Set up a designated room for dressing changes, ensuring it is cleaned daily. The dressing table must be disinfected after each use. If needed, dressings can be applied at the patient's bedside using a clean, disinfected trolley. The trolley should have:

An upper tray with sterile and clean materials (dressing sets, compresses)

A lower tray for contaminated materials (containers for used instruments, sharps disposal, and waste bags)

Preparing for the Procedure

1. Wash Hands or Use Alcohol-based Hand Rub

Before beginning, clean hands thoroughly or disinfect them with an alcohol-based hand rub.

2. Set Up All Materials in a Well-lit Area

If necessary, ask for assistance, especially when dealing with complex wounds.

3. Wear Protective Gear

Depending on the wound's condition, consider wearing protective glasses, particularly if there is a risk of projection from an oozing wound. Always start with clean wounds before moving to those that may be infected.

4. Patient Comfort and Cooperation

Position the patient comfortably while ensuring their privacy throughout the procedure. Always explain the process to the patient and obtain their cooperation.

5. Instruments and Gloves

Change instruments or gloves between patients to prevent cross-contamination.

Procedure for Removing an Old Dressing and Cleaning the Wound

1. Observe the Wound

Examine the wound for any signs of infection (e.g., redness, swelling, discharge). If such signs are present, check for any systemic signs of infection, such as fever or chills.

2. Cleaning the Wound

First, wash hands or disinfect them with alcohol-based hand rub.

Put on non-sterile gloves and gently remove the old dressing. If it sticks to the wound, loosen it using sterile saline or water.

Inspect the used dressing for signs of infection such as greenish discoloration or a foul odor, which indicates a possible infection.

Discard the used dressing and gloves in the appropriate waste container.

3. Wound Assessment

Necrosis (Black Area): Indicates infected or dead tissue.

Yellow/Green Area: Signifies the presence of pus and infected tissue.

Red Area: Granulating tissue, which suggests the wound is healing.

Pink Area: Represents epithelialization, the final stage of wound healing.

In the case of sutured wounds, if there is any evidence of infection, remove the sutures to prevent the spread of infection. Indicators of infection include painful, swollen edges or pus drainage between sutures.

4. Disinfection and Dressing

After inspecting the wound, disinfect it using sterile saline or water.

Dry the wound with a sterile compress.

For sutured wounds or clean open wounds, apply sterile compresses. For infected wounds, use antiseptic solutions like povidone iodine.

Dress the wound with a sterile dressing, ensuring it covers the wound and extends a few centimeters beyond the edges.

Secure the dressing with adhesive tape or a bandage.

Subsequent Dressing and Care

1. Aftercare

Safely dispose of any sharp objects in a sharps container.

Soak reusable instruments in disinfectant and wash hands again.

Clean sutured wounds and change dressings regularly, based on the wound's condition:

Clean sutured wound: Dress every 5 days if the wound remains clean and painless.

Infected sutured wound: Dress daily and remove any pus.

Open wounds: Clean and dress daily, especially if granulating.

Granulating wounds: Change dressings every 2-3 days unless granulation is hypertrophic, in which case apply corticosteroids.

2. Healing Process

The goal of dressing is to facilitate wound healing without complications. For a simple wound, initial cleaning, exploration, and excision (if necessary) should be performed while respecting aseptic procedures. Immediate suturing may be necessary for fresh, clean wounds (less than 6 hours old), while delayed suturing is indicated for contaminated or older wounds.

3. Wound Management

In cases of infected wounds or significant tissue loss, healing by secondary intention (i.e., the wound heals without suturing) may be necessary. If a wound does not meet the cleanliness criteria for suturing, it should heal naturally or require a skin graft after cleaning.

4. Post-Procedure Wound Monitoring
Monitor the wound for any signs of infection or complications. If systemic infection signs such as fever or chills develop, consider initiating systemic antibiotics.

Figures 1: Basic Instruments

1. Kocher Forceps (Straight, Toothed)
Used for securely clamping tissue or materials, with toothed jaws for a firm grip.

(1a)

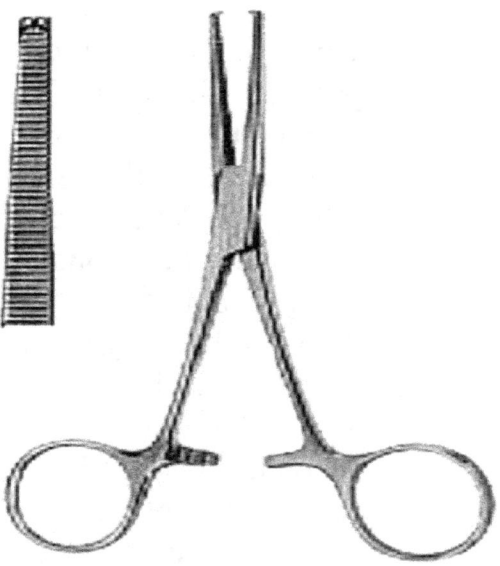

2. Kelly Forceps (Curved, Non-Toothed)
Ideal for clamping blood vessels or tissue, with a curved shape for

better access and non-toothed jaws to reduce tissue damage.

(1b)

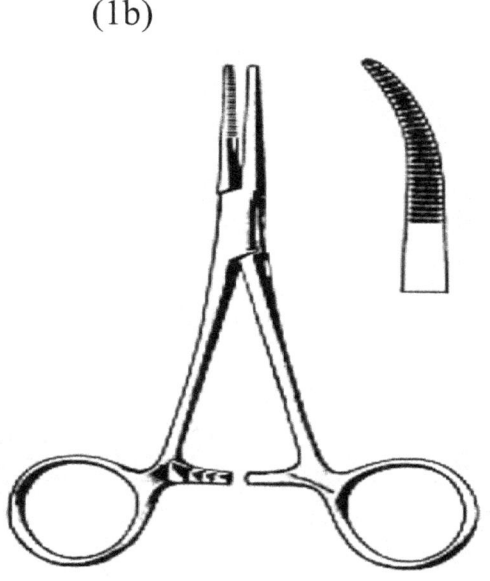

3. Small Artery Forceps (Curved, Non-Toothed)
Designed for clamping smaller vessels or tissue, featuring curved, non-toothed jaws to protect delicate structures.

(1c)

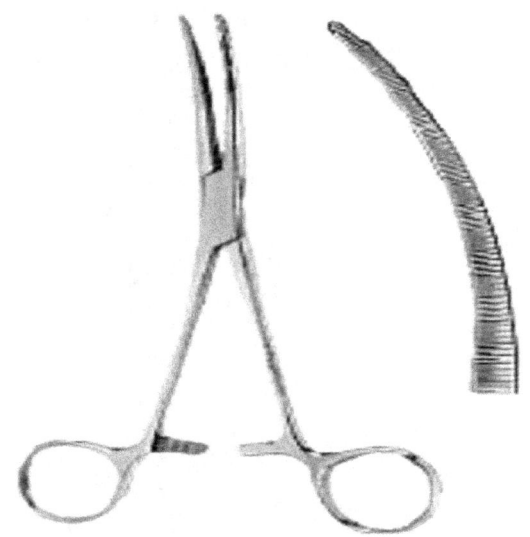

4. Farabeuf Retractor
A tool used to hold back tissues
or organs during procedures.
(1d)

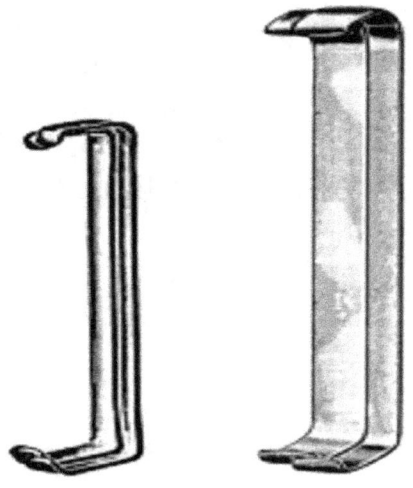

Figures 2: Instrument Handling

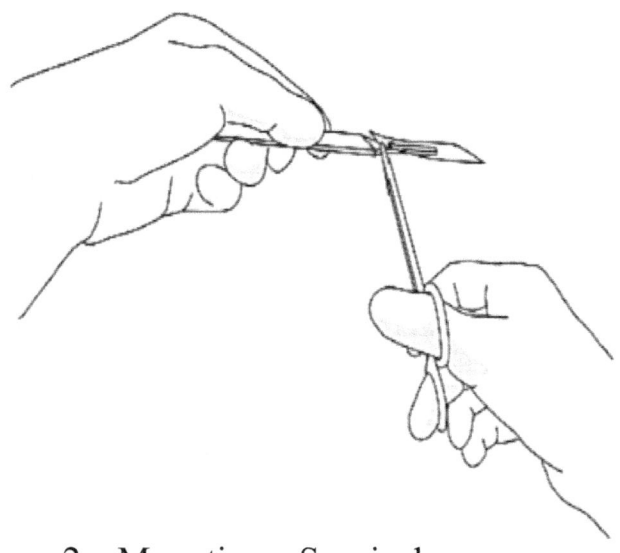

Figure 2a: Mounting a Surgical Blade
Always attach the surgical blade using a needle holder. Ensure that a new blade is used for each procedure.

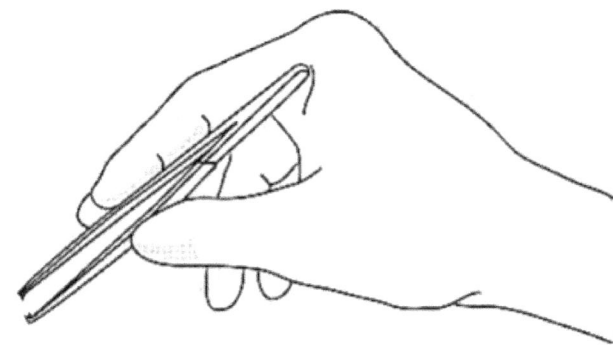

Figure 2b: Proper Use of Dissecting Forceps
Hold dissecting forceps between the thumb and index finger, not in the palm. Use toothed forceps exclusively for handling skin.

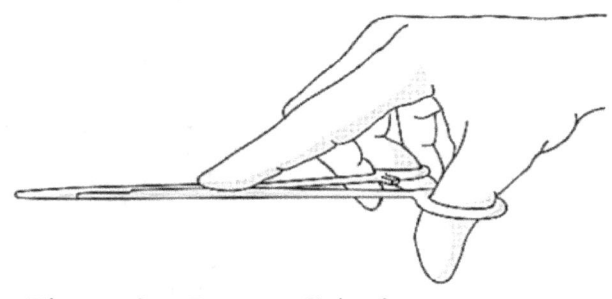

Figure 2c: Proper Grip for Needle Holders or Scissors
Place your thumb and ring finger in the handle loops, using your index finger for stability.

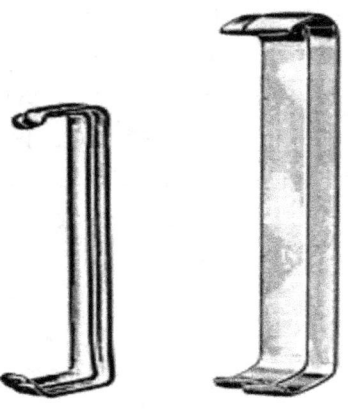

Figure 2d: Small Artery Forceps
Grasp the handle with your thumb and index finger, supported by the middle finger for control.

Figure 3: Wound Debridement
Debridement should be performed conservatively, focusing only on removing

severely damaged or lacerated tissue that is evidently necrotic.

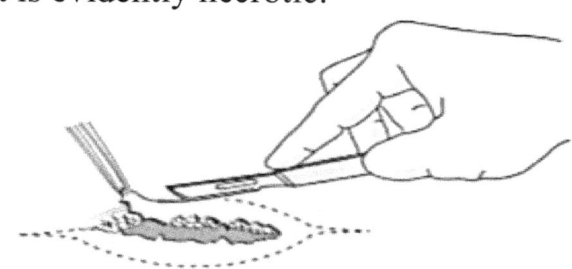

Figure 3a: Debridement of a Contused Wound

Use a scalpel to align irregular wound edges, taking a cautious approach, especially for facial injuries.

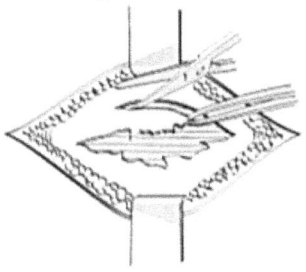

Figure 3b: Aponeurosis Edge Excision

Trim the aponeurosis edges to minimize the risk of necrosis.

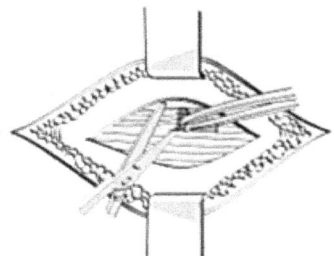

Figure 3c: Removal of Damaged Muscle

Excise severely contused muscle tissue.

Comprehensive Overview of Burn Management: Classification, Evaluation, and Treatment

Definition and Overview

Burns are skin injuries caused by thermal, electrical, chemical, or radiation exposure. These injuries are associated with significant pain and can compromise survival or functionality, depending on the severity and location.

Classification of Burns

Burns are categorized into minor or severe, based on several clinical parameters:

Minor Burns:

Affect less than 10% of body surface area (BSA) in children or 15% in adults.

No associated risk factors.

Severe Burns:

Involve more than 10% of BSA in children or 15% in adults.

Include inhalation injuries, burns caused by chemicals or electricity, and burns on sensitive areas such as the face, hands, joints, or genitalia.

Associated with major trauma or in patients aged under 3 years, over 60 years, or with significant comorbidities.

Burn Evaluation

1. Extent of Burns

The Lund-Browder Table is used to estimate the percentage of BSA affected, adjusted for the patient's age. For example:

A child aged 2 with burns involving the face (8.5%), anterior trunk (13%), and circumferential left upper arm (4%) has a total burn surface area of 27% BSA.

2. Depth of Burns

Burn depth is classified as:

First-degree: Limited to the epidermis; painful erythema without blisters.

Second-degree: Blisters and partial-thickness damage, with varying degrees of healing potential.

Third-degree: Full-thickness damage; often painless due to nerve destruction.

3. Inhalation Injury

Indicators include dyspnea, soot in airways, carbonaceous sputum, or voice hoarseness. These injuries significantly increase mortality risk and require immediate attention.

Treatment of Severe Burns

Initial Management

Airway and Breathing: Ensure airway patency and administer high-flow oxygen, even if SpO_2 is normal.

Circulation: Establish IV access and initiate fluid resuscitation using Ringer's Lactate (RL). For instance:

Administer 20 ml/kg RL within the first hour for stabilization.

Adjust fluids based on the Parkland Formula: 4 ml/kg x %BSA for the first 24 hours, with half given in the first 8 hours.

Analgesia: Administer morphine subcutaneously (0.2 mg/kg) for effective pain relief.

Wound Management: Remove non-adherent clothing and decontaminate chemical burns with copious water irrigation.

General Management in the First 48 Hours

Fluid and Electrolyte Balance: Monitor urine output (target: 1–2 ml/kg/hour) and systolic arterial pressure (SAP).

Avoid fluid overload while ensuring adequate perfusion.
Respiratory Support:
Provide humidified oxygen and chest physiotherapy. Escharotomies may be required in cases of restrictive burns affecting the chest.
Nutritional Support:
Begin enteral feeding within 8 hours of admission, prioritizing high-calorie and high-protein diets to meet the elevated metabolic demands.
Infection Control and Local Treatment
Infection Prevention:
Use aseptic techniques during dressing changes and isolate patients with fresh burns. Administer prophylactic tetanus vaccination.
Topical and Systemic Antibiotics:
For local infections, apply silver sulfadiazine, avoiding use in neonates.
Treat systemic infections with IV cefazolin and oral ciprofloxacin based on clinical severity.
Additional Measures
Physiotherapy: Initiate from Day 1 to prevent contractures.

Pain and Psychological Management: Address insomnia and depression to improve recovery outcomes.

Surgical Intervention: Deep or non-healing burns may require excision and grafting.

Evidence-Based Case Analysis

Case Example:

A 5-year-old child presents with circumferential burns involving 30% of BSA (anterior trunk, both arms, and perineum). Clinical interventions include:

1. Fluid Resuscitation: Administered as per Parkland formula with continuous monitoring of SAP and urine output.
2. Nutritional Management: Early nasogastric feeding initiated to meet metabolic requirements.
3. Wound Care: Sterile dressing changes every 48 hours to minimize infection risk.
4. Physiotherapy: Instituted on Day 1 to maintain joint mobility.

Monitoring and Frequency of Care

Routine Monitoring: Assess the patient every 48 hours to track progress and detect potential complications.

Daily Monitoring: Increase frequency to daily assessments if there is a suspected superinfection or if the patient is in high-risk areas, such as the perineum.

Ischemia Risk

During the initial 48 hours, distal ischemia of the burned limb is the primary concern. Monitoring for ischemic signs should include:

Cyanosis or pallor of the affected extremity

Dysaesthesia, hyperalgesia, or impaired capillary refill

Additionally, daily monitoring should address:

Pain levels

Bleeding

Healing progress

Infection signs

Emergency Surgical Interventions

1. Escharotomy: Performed on circumferential burns to prevent ischemia, especially for extremities or neck areas that may restrict blood flow or impair respiratory function.

2. Tracheotomy: Indicated when airway obstruction occurs due to edema, particularly in cases of deep cervicofacial burns. This procedure can be conducted through a burned area.

3. Tarsorrhaphy: Required in cases of ocular or deep eyelid burns to protect the eyes and prevent further damage.

4. Surgical Care for Associated Injuries: Involves managing fractures or visceral injuries in addition to burn care.

Burn Surgery

Excision-Grafting: For deep burns, excision of necrotic tissue (eschar) followed by grafting with autografts (thin skin) typically occurs between days 5-6 of the burn. This procedure carries a significant bleeding risk, and no more than 15% of the body surface area (BSA) should be involved in a single surgery.

Sloughing, Granulation, and Reepithelialization: If early excision-grafting is not feasible, a slower healing process of sloughing, followed by granulation and reepithelialization, is initiated.

This process is more time-consuming, lasting over a month, and has a higher infection risk.

Pain Management

General Management: Pain intensity varies, so regular assessments are crucial. A simple verbal scale (SVS) can be used for children over 5 years and adults, while the FLACC or NFCS scales are preferred for younger children.

Morphine is the primary treatment for moderate to severe pain. Due to the high potential for developing tolerance, the dosage often needs to be increased. Adjuvant therapies, such as massage therapy or psychotherapy, can complement analgesics.

Types of Pain:

Continuous Pain:

Moderate pain: Paracetamol (PO) + tramadol (PO)

Moderate to severe pain: Paracetamol (PO) + sustained-release morphine (PO)

Acute Pain (during procedures): Additional analgesics are given to manage acute pain experienced during care procedures.

Chronic Pain (during rehabilitation): For minor burns or those requiring less invasive treatments, oral pain medications may suffice. In severe burns, where oral absorption is limited in the first 48 hours, morphine is administered subcutaneously (SC).

Pain Management during Treatment:

Mild to moderate pain: 60-90 minutes before care, administer tramadol (PO).

Moderate to severe pain:

Immediate-release morphine (PO): Initial dose 0.5-1 mg/kg; effective dose generally 1 mg/kg.

Morphine (SC): Initial dose 0.2-0.5 mg/kg; effective dose usually 0.5 mg/kg.

Adjust morphine doses based on pain intensity (SVS). If pain intensity remains high (SVS ≥ 2), increase the dose by 25-50%. If pain is unmanageable, consider performing the procedure under general anesthesia in the operating room.

Pain Management during Dressing Changes

Patient Monitoring: Continuous monitoring of consciousness

level, respiratory rate (RR), heart rate, and oxygen saturation (SpO2) every 15 minutes for the first hour post-dressing change, followed by routine checks.

Dose Adjustments: After assessing pain levels, morphine doses should be adjusted:

If SVS score is 0 or 1, maintain the current dose.

If SVS score ≥ 2, increase the dose by 25-50%.

Use of Alternative Analgesics

In cases where morphine is unavailable, or general anesthesia cannot be administered, low doses of ketamine (0.5-1 mg/kg IM) can be added to enhance pain relief, in combination with paracetamol and tramadol.

Wound Care

Dressings: Use silver sulfadiazine for patients over 2 months and adults, or petrolatum gauze for burns that do not require more intensive treatment (e.g., first-degree burns).

Pain: For mild to moderate burns, paracetamol and tramadol are usually sufficient to manage pain.

Footnotes

The use of outdated techniques like the "naked burn patient under a mosquito net" or water immersion therapy should be avoided in modern practice.

Cutaneous Abscess

A cutaneous abscess is a localized collection of pus within the dermis or subcutaneous tissues, typically caused by Staphylococcus aureus. The abscess presents as a red, painful, shiny nodule, which may or may not show fluctuance. It is often associated with surrounding cellulitis, regional lymphadenopathy, and fever. Complications include osteomyelitis, septic arthritis, and septic shock.

Clinical Features

Local Symptoms: Painful, red, and swollen area with or without fluctuance.

Systemic Symptoms: Fever and regional adenopathy may occur.

Complications: Osteomyelitis, septic arthritis, septic shock.

Investigations

Radiography: In cases of suspected osteomyelitis or septic arthritis, radiography can provide additional diagnostic information.

Treatment

Incision and Drainage (I&D): The primary treatment for a cutaneous abscess is surgical incision and drainage under sterile conditions.

Indications for Surgical Referral: Abscesses located in critical areas such as the anterior neck, central face, perirectal region, hands, or those near major blood vessels (e.g., femoral artery). Additionally, abscesses that involve joints and bones require surgical consultation.

Antibiotic Therapy: Consider antibiotics if systemic infection signs are present, if there is extensive surrounding cellulitis, or if the patient has immunosuppressive conditions such as diabetes. Refer to Erysipelas and Cellulitis, Chapter 4 for detailed antibiotic recommendations.

Equipment for I&D

Sterile Instruments: Sterile scalpel, sterile non-toothed curved artery forceps (e.g., Kelly type), sterile gloves, and antiseptic solution.

Anesthesia:
For small abscesses (<5 cm), local anesthesia using 1% lidocaine (without epinephrine) is sufficient.
Larger abscesses or those in children may require procedural sedation or general anesthesia (e.g., ketamine IM at 10 mg/kg).
Technique
Incision: Hold the scalpel between the thumb and middle finger, with the index finger pressing on the handle. Position the scalpel perpendicular to the skin, and make a single incision along the long axis of the abscess. Ensure the incision is large enough for finger exploration.
Exploration: Use the index finger to explore the abscess cavity, break down loculi, and evacuate pus. Assess the extent, depth, and location relative to underlying structures (e.g., arteries, bone). In cases of bone involvement, seek surgical advice.
Washing: Flush the cavity with 0.9% sodium chloride to cleanse the area.
Drainage: For deeper abscesses, insert a drain or gauze wick,

securing it to the incision edge with a single suture. Remove the drain after 3-5 days.

Pyomyositis

Pyomyositis is a bacterial infection of the muscle, most commonly caused by Staphylococcus aureus. It frequently affects the muscles of the limbs and torso. Infections may involve multiple sites simultaneously. Delay in treatment can lead to severe complications and increased mortality.

Risk Factors

Immunosuppression

Malnutrition

Trauma

Injection drug use

Clinical Features

Local Symptoms: Exquisite muscle tenderness and swelling, often presenting with a "woody" texture upon palpation.

Systemic Symptoms: Fever and regional adenopathy.

Specific Signs: In pyomyositis of the psoas muscle, the patient may present with a flexed hip and pain on hip extension, resembling appendicitis in cases of right-sided involvement.

Investigations
POCUS: Useful for characterizing the abscess and ruling out deep venous thrombosis.
Radiography: May reveal foreign bodies, signs of osteomyelitis, or osteosarcoma.
Treatment
Immobilization: Immobilize the affected limb to reduce movement-induced stress on the infected muscle.
Antibiotics: Systemic antibiotic therapy is indicated for all cases. Refer to Erysipelas and Cellulitis, Chapter 4 for specific antibiotic regimens.
Analgesia: Adapt pain management to the patient's level of discomfort (see Pain, Chapter 1).
Surgical Treatment
Incision and Drainage: Follow the protocol for abscess drainage (as in cutaneous abscess treatment), but note that muscle abscesses are often deeper and may require aspiration with a large-bore needle. Surgical drainage is necessary even if aspiration removes pus.

Incision Technique: Make a generous incision over the abscess site, carefully dissecting through muscle layers using non-toothed forceps or rounded scissors. If the abscess is deep, referral to a surgeon may be necessary.

Drainage: After pus evacuation, insert a large drain and secure it with a suture. The drain should be removed after 5 days.

Leg Ulcers

Leg ulcers are chronic open wounds that may result from a variety of underlying conditions, such as vascular insufficiency, infections, metabolic disorders (e.g., diabetes), and trauma.

Aetiologies

Vascular: Venous and arterial insufficiency

Infectious: Leprosy, ulcer (caused by Mycobacterium), phagedenic ulcer, yaws, syphilis

Parasitic: Dracunculiasis (Guinea worm disease), leishmaniasis

Metabolic: Diabetes

Traumatic: Trauma exacerbating pre-existing conditions

Clinical Management

Initial Care: Bathe the leg in NaDCC solution for 10-15

minutes, then rinse with boiled water. Remove necrotic or fibrinous tissue with compresses or scalpel excision.

Topical Treatment:
Clean ulcers with minimal discharge: Apply 10% povidone iodine and vaseline.
Dirty ulcers with minimal discharge: Use silver sulfadiazine in a controlled manner to avoid systemic side effects.
Oozing ulcers: Apply diluted 10% povidone iodine, followed by saline rinse.
Dressing: Cover with a dry, sterile dressing.

Systemic Treatment
Antibiotics: Indicated in cases of secondary infections, phagedenic ulcers, or when there is evidence of systemic infection.
Doxycycline (adults 200 mg daily, children 4 mg/kg daily) or Metronidazole (adults 500 mg three times daily) can be used, adjusted for patient age and clinical response.
Complementary Therapy: Elevate legs in cases of venous insufficiency, and consider skin grafting for extensive ulcers or those with poor healing potential.

Tetanus Prophylaxis
Ensure appropriate tetanus prophylaxis in cases with high risk of contamination.

Necrotising Soft Tissue Infections

Necrotising infections of the skin and soft tissues, such as necrotising cellulitis and fasciitis, are severe, life-threatening conditions that require immediate intervention.

Risk Factors
- Immunosuppression
- Diabetes
- Trauma
- Malnutrition
- Advanced age

Clinical Features
Early Signs: Erythema, swelling, and disproportionate pain.
Late Signs: Necrosis, hemorrhagic blisters, crepitus, and fetid odor (gas gangrene).
Systemic Signs: Fever, tachycardia, hypotension, and signs of severe sepsis.

Diagnostic Workup
Radiography: May show gas in the muscles or fascial planes, and can help rule out other conditions like foreign bodies or osteomyelitis.

Blood Tests: Elevated white blood cell count, serum creatinine, or glucose can indicate severe infection.

Treatment

Surgical Management: Rapid debridement, drainage, and excision of necrotic tissue are crucial. Surgical re-evaluation within 24-36 hours is necessary to assess the progression of the infection.

Antibiotic Therapy: High-dose IV antibiotics should be initiated immediately after obtaining cultures. Standard regimens include broad-spectrum agents like clindamycin, meropenem, or vancomycin.

Footnotes:

(a) Cloxacillin powder for injection should be reconstituted with 4 ml of water for injection. For children weighing less than 20 kg, dilute each dose in 5 ml/kg of 0.9% sodium chloride or 5% glucose. For children 20 kg and over, as well as adults, dilute in a 100 ml bag of 0.9% sodium chloride or 5% glucose.

(b) Ceftriaxone powder for injection must be reconstituted with water for injection only. For

IV infusion, dilute each dose in 5 ml/kg of 0.9% sodium chloride or 5% glucose for children under 20 kg. For children weighing 20 kg or more, and adults, dilute in a 100 ml bag of 0.9% sodium chloride or 5% glucose.
(c) For administration, dilute each dose of clindamycin in 5 ml/kg of 0.9% sodium chloride or 5% glucose in children under 20 kg. For children 20 kg and over, as well as adults, dilute in a 100 ml bag of 0.9% sodium chloride or 5% glucose.
(d) Dilute each dose of amoxicillin/clavulanic acid in 5 ml/kg of 0.9% sodium chloride for children under 20 kg. For children 20 kg and over, as well as adults, dilute in a 100 ml bag of 0.9% sodium chloride. Do not use glucose for dilution.

.Venomous Bites and Stings: Clinical Manifestations and Management

Snake Bites and Envenomation

Snake bites are categorized into "dry" and "envenomated" types, with the latter leading to serious complications. The severity of envenomation depends on several factors, including the species, the amount of venom injected, the bite's location, and the age and health of the victim. Children are more vulnerable to severe effects. Head and neck bites pose the highest risk.

Clinical Presentation and Treatment:

1. Dry Bites: These bites show no signs of envenomation. Patients may experience localized pain, but venom has not been injected.

Management: Clean the wound, immobilize the affected limb, and monitor for signs of venom injection. Tetanus prophylaxis should be administered.

2. Envenomated Bites (10-30 minutes post-bite):

Symptoms: Hypotension, excessive salivation, sweating, muscle weakness, and respiratory distress.

Species: Elapids (e.g., cobras, mambas), which cause neurological symptoms including respiratory paralysis.

Treatment: Immediate IV access, administration of antivenom, and pain management.

3. Viperid or Crotalid (e.g., rattlesnakes) Envenomation (30 minutes to 5 hours):
Symptoms: Local swelling, intense pain, and systemic signs like hypotension and respiratory difficulty.
Treatment: Antivenom administration, IV analgesics, and anti-inflammatory medications. Blood clotting tests are essential for monitoring coagulation abnormalities.

4. Late Symptoms (6+ hours):
Signs: Hemorrhagic syndrome with signs such as epistaxis, purpura, and disseminated intravascular coagulation (DIC).
Management: Monitoring of coagulation with blood tests and transfusion if necessary. Surgical intervention for tissue necrosis may be required after stabilization.

5. Asymptomatic Bites:
Management: If no signs of envenomation or coagulation abnormalities are observed, monitor for 12-24 hours. If no changes, discharge the patient.

Scorpion Stings and Envenomation

Scorpion envenomation presents primarily in two forms: neurotoxic and local tissue damage. Neurotoxic symptoms, including muscle spasms, tachycardia, and excessive sweating, are common, especially in children. Severe envenomation is rare but can lead to complications like respiratory failure and shock.

Clinical Presentation and Treatment:

1. General Symptoms: Pain at the sting site, swelling, sweating, and muscle pain.

Management: Supportive care with IV fluids, anti-inflammatory medications, and calcium gluconate for muscle spasms. If severe, antivenom may be used, though it is often poorly tolerated.

2. Severe Symptoms (if envenomation occurs):

Symptoms: Muscle pain, tachycardia, excessive sweating, vomiting, and respiratory difficulties.

Treatment: Antivenom administration is effective only within 2-3 hours post-sting. For seizures, diazepam can be used with caution.

3. Anaphylactic Reaction: Rare, but if it occurs, immediate administration of epinephrine is required. Dosing varies by age:
Children under 6: 0.15 mL
Children 6-12 years: 0.3 mL
Adults: 0.5 mL

Spider Bites and Envenomation

There are two major types of spider envenomation: neurotoxic (e.g., black widow spider) and necrotic (e.g., recluse spider). The latter can cause significant tissue damage.

1. Neurotoxic Syndrome (Black Widow Spider):
Symptoms: Severe muscle pain, tachycardia, sweating, nausea, and vomiting. Symptoms typically resolve spontaneously after 24-48 hours.
Treatment: Pain management and supportive care.

2. Necrotic Syndrome (Recluse Spider):
Symptoms: Localized tissue necrosis, fever, and malaise.
Treatment: Wound care, pain management, and sometimes surgical debridement if necrosis is extensive.

Hymenoptera Stings (Bees, Wasps, Hornets)
Hymenoptera stings commonly cause local pain and swelling. However, severe reactions such as anaphylaxis can occur in some individuals.
Clinical Presentation and Management:
1. Local Reactions:
Symptoms: Pain, swelling, and erythema at the sting site.
Management: Clean the sting site, apply calamine lotion for itching, and administer oral analgesics (e.g., paracetamol).
2. Severe Reactions:
Symptoms: Shock, difficulty breathing, and widespread swelling.
Management: Administer epinephrine intramuscularly. In cases of severe reactions, repeat doses may be needed every 5 minutes. Follow up with IV epinephrine if necessary.
Dental Infections
Dental infections typically arise from inflammation of the dental pulp, with complications ranging from localized abscesses to widespread infections that can extend into the surrounding

tissues, including the cervico-facial region.
Clinical Features and Treatment:
1. Localized Dental Abscess:
Symptoms: Pain around the affected tooth, swelling, and potential pus drainage.
Treatment: Root canal therapy or extraction, along with pain management using paracetamol or ibuprofen.
2. Acute Dento-Alveolar Abscess:
Symptoms: Intense pain, fever, and localized swelling.
Treatment: Drainage and/or tooth extraction, followed by a 5-day course of amoxicillin.
3. Cervico-Facial Infection:
Symptoms: Severe swelling, fever, and possible crepitus in the cervical region, indicating gangrenous cellulitis.
Management: Emergency surgical intervention, high-dose antibiotics, and intensive care support if sepsis develops.

Glossary

1. ABG (Arterial Blood Gas)
A test measuring the levels of oxygen, carbon dioxide, and pH in the blood to assess respiratory function and acid-base balance.

2. ACE Inhibitor (Angiotensin-Converting Enzyme Inhibitor)
A class of drugs that lower blood pressure by inhibiting the enzyme responsible for the conversion of angiotensin I to angiotensin II, a potent vasoconstrictor.

3. Acquired Immunodeficiency Syndrome (AIDS)
A disease caused by HIV that weakens the immune system, making individuals more susceptible to infections and certain cancers.

4. Antibiotic Resistance
The ability of bacteria or other microorganisms to resist the effects of drugs that once killed or inhibited their growth.

5. Angina Pectoris
Chest pain or discomfort caused by reduced blood flow to the heart muscle, often a symptom of coronary artery disease.

6. Arteriosclerosis
A condition in which the blood vessels become thickened, stiff, and less elastic, often leading to high blood pressure and heart disease.

7. Bacterial Meningitis

A severe infection of the protective membranes covering the brain and spinal cord, often caused by bacteria such as Neisseria .

8. Blood Urea Nitrogen (BUN)

A measure of kidney function that quantifies the amount of nitrogen in the blood that comes from urea, a waste product.

9. Bradycardia

A slower-than-normal heart rate, typically defined as fewer than 60 beats per minute in adults.

10. Chronic Obstructive Pulmonary Disease (COPD)

A group of lung diseases, including emphysema and chronic bronchitis, that cause airflow limitation and breathing difficulties.

11. Coronary Artery Disease (CAD)

A condition where the arteries supplying blood to the heart muscle become narrowed or blocked, often leading to heart attacks.

12. CT Scan (Computed Tomography)

A diagnostic imaging technique that uses X-rays and computer processing to create detailed images of internal body structures.

13. Deep Vein Thrombosis (DVT)
A condition in which a blood clot forms in a deep vein, often in the legs, which can lead to complications such as pulmonary embolism.

14. Electrocardiogram (ECG)
A test that records the electrical activity of the heart, helping diagnose heart rhythm problems, heart attacks, and other cardiac conditions.

15. Endotracheal Intubation
A medical procedure where a tube is inserted into the trachea to maintain an open airway during anesthesia or respiratory distress.

16. Heart Failure (HF)
A condition where the heart is unable to pump blood effectively to meet the body's needs, leading to symptoms such as shortness of breath and fatigue.

17. HIV (Human Immunodeficiency Virus)
The virus that causes AIDS, attacking and weakening the immune system by destroying

CD4 cells, which are crucial for immune defense.

18. Hypertension
A condition where blood pressure is consistently higher than normal, increasing the risk of heart disease, stroke, and kidney failure.

19. Inflammatory Bowel Disease (IBD)
Chronic inflammation of the digestive tract, including conditions such as Crohn's disease and ulcerative colitis.

20. Magnetic Resonance Imaging (MRI)
A non-invasive imaging technique that uses powerful magnets and radio waves to create detailed images of organs and tissues.

21. Nephrotic Syndrome
A kidney disorder characterized by excessive protein loss in the urine, causing swelling and an increased risk of infections and blood clots.

22. Outpatient Department (OPD)
A medical facility where patients receive care without being admitted to the hospital, often for

minor conditions or follow-up appointments.

23. Sepsis

A life-threatening condition resulting from the body's response to an infection, causing widespread inflammation, organ dysfunction, and potentially organ failure.

24. Tachycardia

An abnormally fast heart rate, typically defined as more than 100 beats per minute in adults.

25. Ultrasound (US)

A diagnostic imaging technique that uses high-frequency sound waves to create images of the internal structures of the body, especially useful for soft tissue examination.

26. Urinalysis (UA)

A test performed on urine to detect signs of kidney disease, urinary tract infections, or other metabolic conditions.

27. Ventilator

A machine used to assist or replace spontaneous breathing in patients who are unable to breathe independently.

28. Viral Hepatitis

Inflammation of the liver caused by a viral infection, often leading to symptoms like jaundice, fatigue, and abdominal discomfort. Common types include Hepatitis A, B, C, D, and E.

29. White Blood Cell Count (WBC)

A blood test that measures the number of white blood cells in the blood, used to help diagnose infections, inflammation, and certain cancers.

www.ingramcontent.com/pod-product-compliance
Lightning Source LLC
Chambersburg PA
CBHW071016240526
45469CB00006BD/1942